全国高等中医药院校中药学类专业双语规划教材

Bilingual Planned Textbooks for Chinese Materia Medica Majors in TCM Colleges and Universities

中药药剂学实验

Pharmaceutical Experiment of Chinese Materia Medica

（供中药学、药学、药物制剂、制药工程及相关专业使用）

(For Chinese Materia Medica, Pharmacy, Pharmaceutics, Pharmaceutical
Engineering and other related majors)

主　编　李小芳　邱智东

副主编　肖学凤　胡慧玲　崔春利　祝侠丽　尹登科

编　者　（以姓氏笔画为序）

尹登科　（安徽中医药大学）　　兰　卫　（新疆医科大学）

刘　芳　（成都中医药大学）　　刘文龙　（湖南中医药大学）

严国俊　（南京中医药大学）　　李小芳　（成都中医药大学）

肖学凤　（天津中医药大学）　　时　军　（广东药科大学）

邱智东　（长春中医药大学）　　谷满仓　（浙江中医药大学）

张纯刚　（辽宁中医药大学）　　国大亮　（天津中医药大学）

罗　佳　（成都中医药大学）　　胡慧玲　（成都中医药大学）

祝侠丽　（河南中医药大学）　　徐　伟　（长春中医药大学）

崔春利　（陕西中医药大学）　　章津铭　（成都中医药大学）

管咏梅　（江西中医药大学）

秘　书　刘　芳

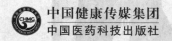

中国健康传媒集团

中国医药科技出版社

内 容 提 要

　　本教材是"全国高等中医药院校中药学类专业双语规划教材"之一。本教材共编写 21 个实验，涵盖传统剂型、普通剂型、新技术与新制剂、开放性实验等多种类型。教材采用中英对应，英文以《中国药典》英文版、《美国药典》《欧洲药典》等为基准，使用文献论文的行文习惯，注重英文翻译的信、达、雅。

　　本教材供中药学、药学、药物制剂、制药工程及相关专业的本科实验教学参考使用，也可作为中药制剂工作者的参考用书。

图书在版编目（CIP）数据

中药药剂学实验：汉英对照 / 李小芳，邱智东主编 . —北京：中国医药科技出版社，2020.12
全国高等中医药院校中药学类专业双语规划教材
ISBN 978-7-5214-1890-3

Ⅰ.①中… Ⅱ.①李… Ⅲ.①中药制剂学－实验－双语教学－中医学院－教材－汉、英 Ⅳ.①R283-33
中国版本图书馆 CIP 数据核字（2020）第 100410 号

美术编辑 陈君杞
版式设计 辰轩文化

出版　**中国健康传媒集团** | 中国医药科技出版社
地址　北京市海淀区文慧园北路甲 22 号
邮编　100082
电话　发行：010-62227427　邮购：010-62236938
网址　www.cmstp.com
规格　889×1194 mm ¹/₁₆
印张　11¼
字数　289 千字
版次　2020 年 12 月第 1 版
印次　2020 年 12 月第 1 次印刷
印刷　三河市万龙印装有限公司
经销　全国各地新华书店
书号　ISBN 978-7-5214-1890-3
定价　41.00 元

获取新书信息、投稿、
为图书纠错，请扫码
联系我们。

近些年随着世界范围的中医药热潮的涌动，来中国学习中医药学的留学生逐年增多，走出国门的中医药学人才也在增加。为了适应中医药国际交流与合作的需要，加快中医药国际化进程，提高来中国留学生和国际班学生的教学质量，满足双语教学的需要和中医药对外交流需求，培养优秀的国际化中医药人才，进一步推动中医药国际化进程，根据教育部、国家中医药管理局、国家药品监督管理局等部门的有关精神，在本套教材建设指导委员会主任委员成都中医药大学彭成教授等专家的指导和顶层设计下，中国医药科技出版社组织全国 50 余所高等中医药院校及附属医疗机构约 420 名专家、教师精心编撰了全国高等中医药院校中药学类专业双语规划教材，该套教材即将付梓出版。

本套教材共计 23 门，主要供全国高等中医药院校中药学类专业教学使用。本套教材定位清晰、特色鲜明，主要体现在以下方面。

一、立足双语教学实际，培养复合应用型人才

本套教材以高校双语教学课程建设要求为依据，以满足国内医药院校开展留学生教学和双语教学的需求为目标，突出中医药文化特色鲜明、中医药专业术语规范的特点，注重培养中医药技能、反映中医药传承和现代研究成果，旨在优化教育质量，培养优秀的国际化中医药人才，推进中医药对外交流。

本套教材建设围绕目前中医药院校本科教育教学改革方向对教材体系进行科学规划、合理设计，坚持以培养创新型和复合型人才为宗旨，以社会需求为导向，以培养适应中药开发、利用、管理、服务等各个领域需求的高素质应用型人才为目标的教材建设思路与原则。

二、遵循教材编写规律，整体优化，紧跟学科发展步伐

本套教材的编写遵循"三基、五性、三特定"的教材编写规律；以"必需、够用"为度；坚持与时俱进，注意吸收新技术和新方法，适当拓展知识面，为学生后续发展奠定必要的基础。实验教材密切结合主干教材内容，体现理实一体，注重培养学生实践技能训练的同时，按照教育部相关精神，增加设计性实验部分，以现实问题作为驱动力来培养学生自主获取和应用新知识的能力，从而培养学生独立思考能力、实验设计能力、实践操作能力和可持续发展能力，满足培养应用型和复合型人才的要求。强调全套教材内容的整体优化，并注重不同教材内容的联系与衔接，避免遗漏和不必要的交叉重复。

三、对接职业资格考试，"教考""理实"密切融合

本套教材的内容和结构设计紧密对接国家执业中药师职业资格考试大纲要求，实现教学与考试、理论与实践的密切融合，并且在教材编写过程中，吸收具有丰富实践经验的企业人员参与教材的编写，确保教材的内容密切结合应用，更加体现高等教育的实践性和开放性，为学生参加考试和实践工作打下坚实基础。

四、创新教材呈现形式，书网融合，使教与学更便捷更轻松

全套教材为书网融合教材，即纸质教材与数字教材、配套教学资源、题库系统、数字化教学服务有机融合。通过"一书一码"的强关联，为读者提供全免费增值服务。按教材封底的提示激活教材后，读者可通过 PC、手机阅读电子教材和配套课程资源（PPT、微课、视频等），并可在线进行同步练习，实时收到答案反馈和解析。同时，读者也可以直接扫描书中二维码，阅读与教材内容关联的课程资源，从而丰富学习体验，使学习更便捷。教师可通过 PC 在线创建课程，与学生互动，开展在线课程内容定制、布置和批改作业、在线组织考试、讨论与答疑等教学活动，学生通过 PC、手机均可实现在线作业、在线考试，提升学习效率，使教与学更轻松。此外，平台尚有数据分析、教学诊断等功能，可为教学研究与管理提供技术和数据支撑。需要特殊说明的是，有些专业基础课程，例如《药理学》等 9 种教材，起源于西方医学，因篇幅所限，在本次双语教材建设中纸质教材以英语为主，仅将专业词汇对照了中文翻译，同时在中国医药科技出版社数字平台"医药大学堂"上配套了中文电子教材供学生学习参考。

编写出版本套高质量教材，得到了全国知名专家的精心指导和各有关院校领导与编者的大力支持，在此一并表示衷心感谢。希望广大师生在教学中积极使用本套教材和提出宝贵意见，以便修订完善，共同打造精品教材，为促进我国高等中医药院校中药学类专业教育教学改革和人才培养做出积极贡献。

全国高等中医药院校中药学类专业双语规划教材
建设指导委员会

数字化教材编委会

主　编　李小芳　邱智东

副主编　肖学凤　胡慧玲　崔春利　祝侠丽　尹登科

编　者　（以姓氏笔画为序）

尹登科（安徽中医药大学）　　兰　卫（新疆医科大学）

刘　芳（成都中医药大学）　　刘文龙（湖南中医药大学）

严国俊（南京中医药大学）　　李小芳（成都中医药大学）

肖学凤（天津中医药大学）　　时　军（广东药科大学）

邱智东（长春中医药大学）　　谷满仓（浙江中医药大学）

张纯刚（辽宁中医药大学）　　国大亮（天津中医药大学）

罗　佳（成都中医药大学）　　胡慧玲（成都中医药大学）

祝侠丽（河南中医药大学）　　徐　伟（长春中医药大学）

崔春利（陕西中医药大学）　　章津铭（成都中医药大学）

管咏梅（江西中医药大学）

秘　书　刘　芳

前　言

本教材是"全国高等中医药院校中药学类专业双语规划教材"之一，为满足新时期中医药行业高素质复合型人才培养的需求，并结合中药药剂学实践性和应用性强的特点而编写。可供中药学、药学、药物制剂、制药工程及相关专业的本科实验教学参考使用，也可为中药制剂工作者参考。本教材共编写 21 个实验，主要特色如下。

1. 教材所涉剂型覆盖面广，注重与理论教材的协调统一。

教材涵盖传统剂型、普通剂型、新技术与新制剂等多种制剂类型，具体包括：煎膏剂、药酒、灸剂等传统剂型；散剂、合剂、糖浆剂、液体药剂、注射剂、软膏剂与乳膏剂、栓剂、丸剂、颗粒剂、片剂、胶囊剂、膜剂等普通剂型；包合物、脂质体、微囊等新技术与新制剂。剂型设计全面，同时设计开放性实验以提高学生的创新思维能力。教材整体编排顺序保持与理论教材的协调统一。

2. 结合执业药师执业要求及企业生产实际，注重常用剂型重点与特色质量检查项目。

强调常用剂型的重点与特色检查项目，如栓剂需检查融变时限，丸剂需检查溶散时限，片剂需检查崩解时限；设计溶出度和释放度实验，将传统固体制剂和新型给药系统主要检查项目进行区分。所有检查项目均根据《中华人民共和国药典》（2020 年版）（以下简称《中国药典》）的有关规定编写。

3. 采用双语体系编写，英文翻译注重信、达、雅。

教材采用中英对应，英文以《中国药典》英文版、《美国药典》《欧洲药典》等为基准，使用文献论文的行文习惯，注重英文翻译的信、达、雅。

本教材是由从事中药药剂学教学与科研工作的骨干教师共同编写。本教材的编写工作得到各编委所在院校的大力支持，在此一并表示感谢。由于编者水平所限，书中难免存在疏漏之处，恳请读者批评指正。

编者
2020 年 5 月

Preface

This textbook is based on the requirements of "Bilingual Planned Textbooks for Chinese Materia Medica Majors in TCM Colleges and Universities" to improve the all-around ability of graduates in the pharmaceutics perspective of Traditional Chinese Medicine, and is compiled in combination with the characteristics of Pharmaceutics of Chinese Materia Medica as a comprehensive applied technology science with strong practicality and applicability. It can be used as a reference for the undergraduate experiment teaching of Chinese Materia Medica, pharmacy, pharmaceutics, pharmaceutical engineering and other related majors, as well as for the workers of Chinese medicine preparation. This textbook contains 21 important laboratories. The main features are as follows:

1. The preparations involved in the textbook cover a wide range and pay attention to the coordination and unification with the theoretical textbook.

The textbook includes traditional preparations, conventional preparations, new technologies and new preparations, open experiments and other preparation types. It specifically includes: traditional preparations such as decoctions, medicinal wine and moxibustion; conventional preparations such as powders, mixture, syrup, liquid medicine, injections, ointments and creams, suppositories, pills, granules, tablets, capsules and membrane; new technologies and new preparations such as inclusion compound, liposomes and microcapsules. The dosage forms are designed comprehensively. At the same time, open experiments are designed to improve students' innovative thinking ability. The overall arrangement order of teaching materials shall be in harmony with the theoretical teaching materials.

2. Combined with the practice requirements of licensed pharmacists and the production practice of enterprises, the textbook focuses on the key points of conventional preparations and characteristic quality inspection items.

It emphasizes the key points and characteristic inspection items of common dosage forms, such as the time limit for suppositories to be checked for melting, pills to be checked for dissolution, tablets to be checked for disintegration; the dissolution and release experiments are designed to distinguish the main inspection items of traditional solid preparation and new drug delivery system. All inspection items are compiled in accordance with *the Pharmacopoeia of the People's Republic of China* (2020) (ChP).

3. This textbook is written in a bilingual system, and English translation focuses on accuracy, fluency and elegance.

The textbook are bilingual in Chinese and English. English is based on the translation of the English version of the ChP, the United States Pharmacopoeia, the European Pharmacopoeia, etc. it uses the writing habits of literature papers and pays attention to the accuracy, fluency and elegance of English translation.

This textbook is written by the experienced professors and scholars in Pharmaceutics of Traditional Chinese Medicine. We would like to acknowledge the kindly support from our editorial board members and their institutes. Due to time restriction and resource limits, omissions may be highly unavoidable. Your valuable opinions and suggestions would be most welcome.

Authors

May 2020

目录 | Contents

实验一　散剂的制备

实验目的

1. **掌握**　一般散剂、含毒性药物散剂、含低共熔混合物散剂的制备方法及其操作要点。
2. **熟悉**　等量递增混合法及其应用。
3. **了解**　散剂的常规质量检查方法。

实验提要

1. 散剂系指饮片或提取物经粉碎、均匀混合制成的粉末状剂型。按给药途径，散剂可分为口服散剂与外用散剂；按药物性质，散剂可分为一般散剂、含毒性药物散剂、含液体药物散剂、含低共熔混合物散剂等。

2. 散剂的制备主要包括药物粉碎、过筛、混合、分剂量、质检、包装等工序。药物粉末粒度的要求：一般内服散剂为细粉，儿科用及外用散剂为最细粉，眼用散剂为极细粉。

3. 混合是散剂制备的关键操作，主要混合方法有研磨混合、搅拌混合与过筛混合。若药物比例相差悬殊，应采用等量递增法混合；若各组分的密度相差悬殊，应将密度小的组分先加入研磨器内，再加入密度大的组分进行混合；若组分的色泽相差悬殊，一般先将色深的组分放入研磨器中，再加入色浅的组分进行混合。

4. 对于小剂量毒剧药物散剂，常添加一定比例的赋形剂制成稀释散，亦称倍散。处方中若含少量低共熔成分，一般先使之产生共熔，再用其他成分吸收混合制成散剂。

实验器材

1. **仪器**　天平、研钵、手摇筛等。
2. **试药**　滑石、甘草、朱砂、麝香草酚、薄荷油、薄荷脑、樟脑、水杨酸、氧化锌、升华硫、淀粉、硼酸、滑石粉、硫酸阿托品、乳糖、胭脂红等。

实验操作步骤

（一）益元散的制备

【处方】

滑石	30.0g
甘草	5.0g
朱砂	1.5g

【制法】 以上三味，滑石、甘草粉碎成细粉，朱砂水飞成极细粉，与上述粉末配研，过筛，混匀。按每包 3g 分装，即得。

实验流程图如图 1-1 所示。

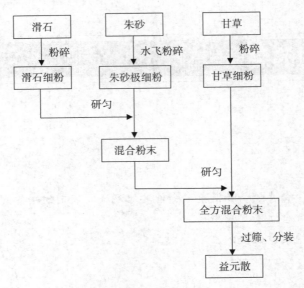

图 1-1　益元散的制备流程图

【性状】本品为浅粉红色粉末，手捻有润滑感，味甜。

【功能与主治】消暑利湿。用于感受暑湿、身热心烦、口渴喜饮、小便赤短等症。

【用法与用量】调服或煎服，一次 6g，一日 1~2 次。

【注意事项】加入朱砂前研钵应预先用少量滑石粉研磨以饱和其表面能。朱砂极细粉应先与滑石粉混匀，以免朱砂极细粉被甘草粉末吸附而"咬色"。朱砂与滑石粉宜采用打底套色法混合。方中各药混合时均应遵循等量递增原则混合。

（二）痱子粉的制备

【处方】

麝香草酚	0.6g	薄荷油	0.6ml
薄荷脑	0.6g	樟脑	0.6g
水杨酸	1.4g	氧化锌	6.0g
升华硫	4.0g	淀粉	10.0g
硼酸	8.6g	滑石粉	加至100g

【制法】取麝香草酚、薄荷脑、樟脑研磨形成低共熔混合物，与薄荷油混匀。另将水杨酸、氧化锌、升华硫、硼酸、淀粉研磨混合，用混合细粉吸收低共熔混合物，最后按等量递增法加入滑石粉研匀，使成100g，过七号筛，即得。

实验流程图如图 1-2 所示。

【性状】本品为白色粉末，手捻有润滑感。

【功能与主治】散风祛湿、清凉止痒。用于汗疹、痱毒、湿疮痛痒。

【用法与用量】外用，撒布患处。一日 1~2 次。

【注意事项】

（1）痱子粉属于含低共熔混合物的散剂，处方中麝香草酚、薄荷脑、樟脑可形成低共熔混合物。制备时先将共熔成分混合使其共熔，与薄荷油混匀后，再用其余混合粉末吸收低共熔物。制备过程中需采用等量递增法（配研法），以利于药物细粉混合均匀。

（2）为保证微生物限度符合规定，制备时应先将滑石粉、氧化锌于 150℃ 干热灭菌 1 小时，淀粉 105℃ 烘干后备用。

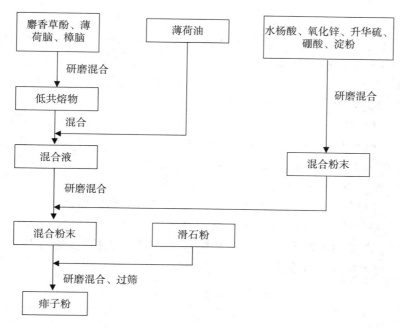

图 1-2　痱子粉的制备流程图

（三）硫酸阿托品散的制备

【处方】

硫酸阿托品	0.25g
乳糖	24.50g
胭脂红乳糖	0.25g

【制法】取乳糖适量，置研钵中研磨，使研钵饱和后倾出，将硫酸阿托品与胭脂红乳糖置研钵中研匀，再以等量递增法逐渐加入乳糖，研匀，待色泽一致后，分装，每包 0.1g。

实验流程图如图 1-3 所示。

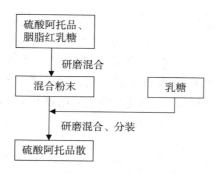

图 1-3　硫酸阿托品散的制备流程图

【性状】本品为淡红色粉末。

【适应证】本品为抗胆碱药，常用于胃肠痉挛疼痛等。

【用法与用量】口服，疼痛时一次 1 包。

【注意事项】胭脂红为着色剂，着色后便于观察散剂的均匀性和不同稀释度散剂间及其与原药的区别。胭脂红乳糖的制法为：取胭脂红 0.1g，置研钵中加入 90% 乙醇 1~2ml，研磨使溶解，再按等量递增法加入乳糖 9.9g，研匀，50~60℃ 干燥，过筛即得。

（四）散剂的质量检查

1. 粒度　除另有规定外，化学药局部用散剂和用于烧伤或严重创伤的中药局部用散剂及儿科用散剂，照下述方法检查，应符合规定。

检查法 除另有规定外，取供试品10g，精密称定，照粒度和粒度分布测定法（通则0982 单筛分法）测定。化学药散剂通过七号筛（中药通过六号筛）的粉末重量，不得少于95%。

2. 外观均匀度 取供试品适量，置光滑纸上，平铺约5cm²，将其表面压平，在明亮处观察，应色泽均匀，无花纹与色斑。

3. 水分 中药散剂照水分测定法（通则0832）测定，除另有规定外，不得过9.0%。

4. 干燥失重 化学药和生物制品散剂，除另有规定外，取供试品，照干燥失重测定法（通则0831）测定，在105℃干燥至恒重，减失重量不得过2.0%。

5. 装量差异 单剂量包装的散剂，照下述方法检查，应符合规定。

检查法 除另有规定外，取供试品10袋（瓶），分别精密称定每袋（瓶）内容物的重量，求出内容物的装量与平均装量。每袋（瓶）装量与平均装量相比较［凡有标示装量的散剂，每袋（瓶）装量应与标示装量相比较］，按表1-1中的规定，超出装量差异限度的散剂不得多于2袋（瓶），并不得有1袋（瓶）超出装量差异限度的1倍。

表 1-1　散剂装量差异限度

平均装量或 标示装量	装量差异限度 （中药、化学药）	装量差异限度 （生物制品）
0.1g 及 0.1g 以下	±15%	±15%
0.1g 以上至 0.5g	±10%	±10%
0.5g 以上至 1.5g	±8%	±7.5%
1.5g 以上至 6.0g	±7%	±5%
6.0g 以上	±5%	±3%

凡规定检查含量均匀度的化学药和生物制品散剂，一般不再进行装量差异的检查。

6. 装量 除另有规定外，多剂量包装的散剂，照最低装量检查法（通则0942）检查，应符合规定。

7. 无菌 除另有规定外，用于烧伤［除程度较轻的烧伤（Ⅰ度或浅Ⅱ度外）］、严重创伤或临床必须无菌的局部用散剂，照无菌检查法（通则1101）检查，应符合规定。

8. 微生物限度 除另有规定外，照非无菌产品微生物限度检查：微生物计数法（通则1105）和控制菌检查法（通则1106）及非无菌药品微生物限度标准（通则1107）检查，应符合规定。凡规定进行杂菌检查的生物制品散剂，可不进行微生物限度检查。

 思考题

1. 等量递增混合的原则是什么？

2. 低共熔现象的含义是什么？在处方中常见的低共熔成分有哪些？怎样制备含低共熔混合物的散剂？

3. 制备稀释散时，如何根据用药剂量确定稀释倍数？

题库

注：本书中所提"通则"均出自《中国药典》2020年版。

Experiment 1 Preparation of Powders

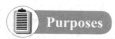 **Purposes**

1. To master the preparation methods and operation points of general powders, powders with toxic drug and eutectic mixture.
2. To be familiar with the mixed method of equivalent increments and its application.
3. To understand the routine quality inspection methods for powders.

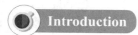 **Introduction**

1. Powders are defined as a dosage form composed of a mixture of decoction pieces or extractions reduced to a finely divided state. According to the modes of administration, powders can be divided into oral powders and topical powders; according to the nature of the ingredients, powders can be divided into general powders, powders with toxic drug, powders with liquid drug, powders with eutectic mixture and so on.

2. The preparation of powders mainly includes procedures of comminution of drugs, sieving, mixing, dosing, quality inspection and packaging. The particle size for oral powders is fine, for pediatric and topical powders is very fine, and for ophthalmic powders is extremely fine.

3. Mixing is the critical process for the preparation of powders. The main mixing methods include trituration, stirring and sifting. When a small amount of ingredient is to be mixed with a large amount of ingredient, the equivalent incremental method is used to ensure the uniform distribution of the ingredients. When the density difference between two ingredients is large, the low-density ingredient should be added into the grinding container first, followed by the high-density ingredient. When the color difference is obvious, the dark color ingredient should be added to the grinding container first, followed by the light color ingredient.

4. For small-dose poisonous drug powders, a certain proportion of excipients are often added to make diluted powders, also known as diluted powders. If the formula contains a small amount of eutectic ingredients, it is generally first caused to eutectic, and then absorbed and mixed with other ingredients to make powders.

Equipments and Materials

1. **Equipments** Balance, mortar, hand sieve, etc.
2. **Materials** Talc, licorice, cinnabar, thymol, peppermint oil, menthol, camphor, salicylic acid, zinc oxide, sublimation sulfur, starch, boric acid, talcum powder, atropine sulfate, lactose, carmine, etc.

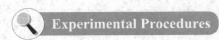 **Experimental Procedures**

（Ⅰ）Preparation of Yiyuan Powders

【Formula】

Talc   30.0g

Licorice   5.0g

Cinnabar   1.5g

【Preparation】Above three drugs, triturate talc and licorice are crushed to the fine powders separately. Cinnabar is to triturated extremely fine by method of water fly smash. Grind the above powder with equivalent incremental method, sieve and mix. Divide and package the final powders 3g per bag.

Experiment flow chart (Figure 1−1):

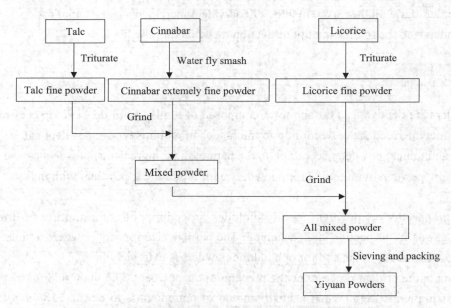

Figure 1−1   **The preparation flow chart of Yiyuan Powders**

【Characters】This product is a light pink powder with sweet taste, and a sense of lubrication by hand twisting.

【Functions and Indications】Clear heat and dampness. It is used to feel hot and humid, upset and hot, thirsty and drink, and short urine.

【Usage and Dosage】Transfer or decoction. 6g at a time, 1~2 times a day.

【Considerations】Before adding cinnabar, add a small amount of talc into the mortar and grind to saturate its surface energy first. Mix the powders of cinnabar and talc first to prevent cinnabar powder from being absorbed by licorice powder. Mix the cinnabar and talc by the "backing and registering" method. Blend all the powders following the principle of equal amount.

（Ⅱ）Preparation of Anti-rash Powders

【Formula】

Thymol	0.6g	Peppermint oil	0.6ml
Menthol	0.6g	Camphor	0.6g
Salicylic acid	1.4g	Zinc oxide	6.0g
Sublimation sulfur	4.0g	Starch	10.0g

Boric acid   8.6g   Talcum powder   Add to 100g

【Preparation】Grind thymol, menthol and camphor to form a eutectic liquid then mix with peppermint oil. Grind and mix the powder of salicylic acid, zinc oxide, sublimated sulfur, boric acid and starch which is used to absorb the eutectic liquid. Finally, add talcum powder by equivalent incremental method to the total amount to 100g and pass the powder mass through the No.7 sieve to get the final product.

Experiment flow chart (Figure 1–2):

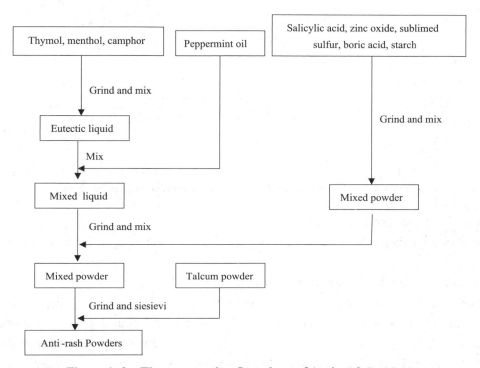

Figure 1–2   The preparation flow chart of Anti-rash Powders

【Characters】This product is a white powder with a sense of lubrication by hand twisting.

【Functions and Indications】Remove wind and dampness, cool and relieve itching. Used for sweat rash, rash, itching.

【Usage and Dosage】Appropriate amount for external use, rub the affected area. 1~2 times a day.

【Considerations】

(1) Anti-rash powders is a powder containing eutectic liquid. In the formula, thymol, menthol and camphor can form eutectic liquid. During the preparation, mix the eutectics first which can form eutectic liquid, and then mix with peppermint oil. Absorb eutectic liquid with remaining powder. In the preparation process, the equivalent incremental method (geometric dilution) is needed to facilitate the uniform mixing of the fine powder.

(2) In order to ensure that the microbial limit meets the requirements, talcum powder and zinc oxide should be sterilized at 150°C for 1h under dry heat, and starch should be dried at 105°C for future use.

（Ⅲ）Preparation of Atropine Sulfate Powders

【Formula】

Atropine sulfate   0.25g

Lactose   24.50g

Carmine lactose   0.25g

【Preparation】Take an appropriate amount of lactose, grind it in a mortar, saturate the mortar, pour it out. Then, mix atropine sulfate with carmine-dyed lactose in the mortar, and grind the obtained mixture. Add lactose by equivalent incremental method. After the color is consistent, divide and package the powders 0.1g per bag to get the final product.

Experiment flow chart (Figure 1–3):

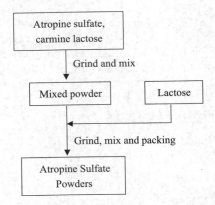

Figure 1–3   The preparation flow chart of Atropine Sulfate Powders

【Characters】This product is light red powder.

【Indications】This product is an anticholinergic drug, commonly used for gastrointestinal cramps and pain.

【Usage and Dosage】Oral, 1 sachet at the time of pain.

【Considerations】Carmine is a colorant. Dyeing with carmine is helpful to observe the uniformity of mixture and differences between powders of the different dilution degrees and original drugs. Preparation of carmine-dyed lactose: dissolve 0.1g carmine into 1~2ml of 90% ethanol in the mortar. Add the lactose 9.9g by equivalent incremental method and grind to uniform. Dry the powder at 50~60°C and pass through the sieve to get the final product.

(Ⅳ) Quality Inspection of Powders

1. Particle size   Unless otherwise specified, powders for topical use, the powders of chemical drugs used for burn or severe trauma, as well as the powders of Chinese medicine for paediatric use, should comply with the following requirements.

Inspection method: Unless otherwise specified, weigh accurately about 10g of the powder. Carry out the determination of particle size and particle size distribution (General rule 0982, single screening). Not less than 95% of the powder should pass though the sieve (No. 7 sieve for powders of chemical drugs, and No. 6 for those of Chinese medicine).

2. Uniformity of appearance   Inspection method: Spread evenly a sufficient quantity of powder in an area of about $5cm^2$ on a piece of smooth paper, press the surface evenly, and observe the powder under a bright light. It should be uniform in coloration with no discolorations and colour stains.

3. Determination of water for Chinese medicinal powder   Carry out the determination of water (General rule 0832). The powders should contain not more than 9.0 percent of water, unless otherwise specified.

4. Loss on drying   For chemical drug powder and biological product powder, unless otherwise specified, carry out the test for loss on drying (General rule 0831). Loss on drying to constant weight at 105°C should be not more than 2.0%.

5. Weight variation The weight variation of powders packaged in single-dose should comply with the requirements in the Table 1-1.

Table 1-1 Weight variation limit for powder

Average or labelled weight	Weight variation limit (Chinese medicine or chemical drug powders)	Weight variation limit (Biological product powders)
0.1g or less	±15%	±15%
More than 0.1g to 0.5g	±10%	±10%
More than 0.5g to 1.5g	±8%	±7.5%
More than 1.5g to 6.0g	±7%	±5%
More than 6.0g	±5%	±3%

Inspection method: Unless otherwise specified, weight accurately the content of each 10 packs (bottles) of powders and calculate the average content weight. Compare the content weight with the average weight (or labelled weight). No more than 2 packs exceed the weight variation limit, and none of them exceed twice the limit. Where the test for content uniformity is specified, the test for weight variation may not be required.

6. Filling Unless otherwise specified, multi-dose packaged powders should comply with the test of minimum fill (General rule 0942).

7. Sterility Unless otherwise specified, powders used for burn except minor burn (1st or minor 2nd degree), severe trauma or powders for topical application required to be sterile in clinic should comply with the sterility test (General rule 1101).

8. Microbial limit Unless otherwise specified, powders should comply with the requirements of microbiological examination of nonsterile products; microbial enumeration tests (General rule 1105). microbiological examination of nonsterile products: test for specified microorganisms (General rule 1106) and microbiological acceptance criteria of nonsterile pharmaceutical products (General rule 1107). Where the test for contaminating microorganisms on powders is specified, the microbial limit test may not be required.

 Questions

1. What is the principle of equivalent incremental method?

2. What is the meaning of the eutectic phenomenon? What are the common eutectic ingredients in the prescription? How to prepare powder containing eutectic mixture?

3. How to determine the dilution factor according to the dosage when preparing the diluted powder?

PPT

实验二　中药合剂（口服液）的制备

实验目的

1. **掌握**　中药合剂（口服液）的制备方法、关键操作和注意事项。
2. **熟悉**　中药合剂（口服液）常规质量要求及其检查方法。
3. **了解**　中药合剂（口服液）的分装设备。

实验提要

1. 中药合剂系指中药饮片用水或其他溶剂，采用适宜的方法提取制成的口服液体制剂，单剂量包装者称为"口服液"。中药合剂（口服液）是在传统汤剂基础上改进和发展起来的中药剂型。

2. 特点。中药合剂（口服液）继承了中药汤剂吸收、奏效迅速的优点；同时，无需临用前煎煮，使用方便；作为汤剂的浓缩制品，服用量减少；再通过矫味，口感较易接受；防腐与灭菌包装处理使得中药合剂质量稳定。然而，合剂贮存期间常有少量摇之易散的沉淀出现；相对汤剂合剂不能随症加减；生产工艺相对较为复杂，生产设备、工艺条件要求较高。

3. 中药合剂（口服液）的制备工艺流程如图 2-1 所示。

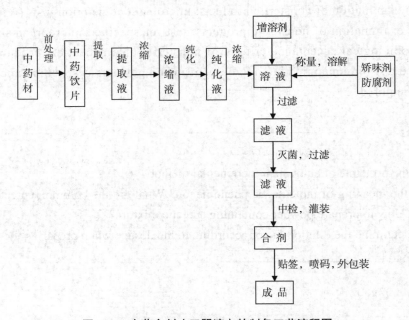

图 2-1　中药合剂（口服液）的制备工艺流程图

（1）中药材前处理　净选 → 水洗 → 润药 → 切制 → 干燥 → 净饮片。

（2）浸提　一般根据药材饮片所含主要化学成分的溶解性等选择适宜浸提方法，常用溶媒为水和乙醇，由于水的极性较大，大多采用加水煎煮法；而对于含有芳香挥发性成分，一般先采用双提法，即先用水蒸气蒸馏法提取挥发性成分，药渣再与处方中其他药材一起加水煎煮。

（3）浓缩　浓缩是指使溶剂蒸发而提高溶液的浓度，在此为脱水操作。中药合剂（口服液）提取液的浓缩程度会影响纯化处理的效果。浓缩应根据处方药物成分的热稳定性，选择适宜的浓缩方法和浓缩条件。一般处方提取液的量往往较大，为接下来的纯化操作带来不便。如，水醇法，当药液浓缩得太稀，要达到一定醇浓度所需要的乙醇量较大，也给醇沉、滤过、回收乙醇等工序造成麻烦。一般浓缩至相对密度约 1.0（50~60℃）或每毫升相当于原药材 1~2g 即可。

（4）纯化　常用纯化方法有高速离心法、水醇法、醇水法、吸附澄清法等。纯化法及其参数的选择（如含醇量、澄清剂用量以及离心的转速等）应以不影响药物成分的含量为指标。

（5）再浓缩　处方中药经过提取纯化后仍需适当浓缩。如经过醇沉精制处理的中药提取液中，含有乙醇和水等溶剂，需要先采用减压浓缩完全回收醇沉上清液中乙醇，继而常压蒸发浓缩除去部分溶剂水，从而达到合剂制备成型的要求。浓缩程度一般以每次服用量在 10~20ml 为宜。

（6）配液　为了使中药合剂具有良好的口感和稳定性，应在洁净、避菌环境中操作，可加入适宜的矫味剂、防腐剂、pH 调节剂、增溶剂及抗氧剂等。合剂若以蔗糖作为矫味剂，含蔗糖量一般不高于 20%（g/ml）。防腐剂山梨酸和苯甲酸钠不得超过 0.3%，羟苯酯类的用量不得超过 0.05%。加入防腐剂的品种和用量应符合国家标准的有关规定，不影响合剂成品的稳定性，并应避免对检验产生干扰，必要时可加入适量的乙醇。

（7）滤过　处方水煎煮提取液的滤过多采用离心机或板框过滤器过滤；纯化处理过的药液和配制的药液多采用板框过滤器和管式离心机分别进行粗滤和精滤（0.22μm）处理。

（8）灌装与灭菌　配制好的药液应尽快用负压式合剂灌装机或灌注式口服液灌装机生产线灌装于无菌的洁净干燥的适宜容器中。单剂量灌装即为口服液，并加盖密封。根据灌装瓶的材质选择适宜灭菌方法，玻璃瓶终端灭菌，先灌装再采用煮沸灭菌、热压灭菌和高温瞬时灭菌等方法。塑料瓶采取精滤液先行灭菌而后灌装，多采取低温间歇灭菌，灭菌后待药液温度降下来后再灌装。

4. 渗漉法属于动态浸出法，在浸提过程中始终能够维持良好浓度梯度，提取效率高，操作简便，室温环境操作，不破坏热敏性成分，故适用于热敏性成分的药材、贵重细料药材及含毒性成分药材的提取。单渗漉法的工艺流程为：药材粉碎 → 润湿 → 装筒 → 排气 → 浸渍 → 渗漉 → 渗漉液。

5. 质量要求。应澄清，在贮存期间不得有发霉、酸败、异物、变色、产生气体或其他变质现象，允许有少量摇之易散的沉淀。一般应检查相对密度、pH 等。单剂量、多剂量灌装合剂均需进行装量及微生物限度检查，均应符合规定。

实验器材

1. **仪器**　电炉（或电磁炉、红外加热炉）、1000ml 规格电热套、渗漉筒、水浴锅、100ml 圆底烧瓶、挥发油分离器、冷凝管、（循环水式或电子）真空泵、布氏漏斗、酒精计、万分之一电子天平、电子天平、pH 计、比重瓶、碾槽（或捣药罐）、1.5ml 塑料离心试管等。

2. **试药**　羌活、防风、苍术、细辛、川芎、白芷、黄芩、甘草、地黄、医用酒精、聚山梨酯 80（也称为吐温 80，tween 80）、山梨酸、蔗糖、蒸馏水。

实验操作步骤

（一）九味羌活口服液的制备
【处方】

| 羌活 30g | 防风 30g | 苍术 30g | 细辛 10g | 川芎 20g |
| 白芷 20g | 黄芩 20g | 甘草 20g | 地黄 20g | |

　　【制法】以上九味，白芷粉碎成粗粉，照流浸膏剂与浸膏剂项下的渗漉法（通则0189），用8倍量70%乙醇作溶剂，浸渍24小时后，进行渗漉，收集渗漉液，备用。羌活、防风、苍术、细辛、川芎加入6倍量水提取挥发油，蒸馏后的水溶液另器收集。药渣与其余黄芩等三味加（10倍/8倍）水煎煮两次，每次1小时，合并煎液，滤过，滤液与上述水溶液合并，浓缩至约180ml，加等量乙醇使沉淀，取上清液与渗漉液合并，回收乙醇，浓缩至相对密度为1.10~1.20（70℃）的清膏，加水稀释至160ml，备用。将20g蔗糖用热溶法制成单糖浆，备用。将挥发油加入0.4ml聚山梨酯80中，再加入少量药液，混匀，然后加入药液、单糖浆以及山梨酸0.2g，混匀，加水至200ml。混匀，分装，灭菌，即得。

　　实验流程图如图2-2所示。

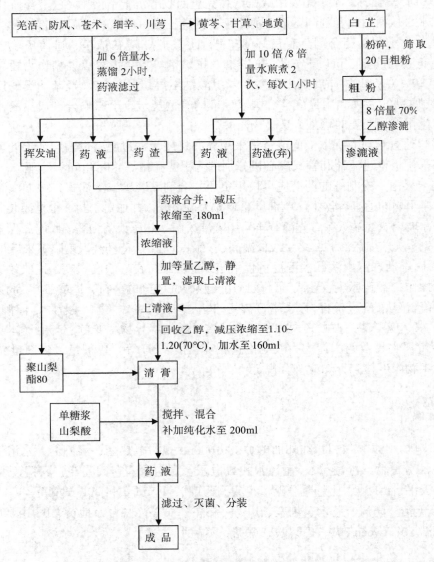

图2-2　九味羌活口服液的制备流程图

　　【性状】本品应为棕褐色的液体。

　　【功能与主治】疏风解表，散寒除湿。用于外感风寒挟湿所致的感冒，症见恶寒、发热、无汗、头重而痛、肢体疼痛。

　　【用法与用量】口服。一次20ml，一日2~3次。

【注意事项】

（1）九味羌活口服液处方中羌活、防风、苍术、细辛和川芎 5 味药材饮片含有较多的挥发性成分，现代研究表明这些药材所含挥发油为其解表的药效成分，故在此采用双提法。

（2）鉴于处方中羌活、防风、苍术、细辛和川芎 5 味药材饮片所含挥发油比重均小于 1，须选用轻油挥发油提取器，为了提高挥发油得率，并防止提取挥发油后药材膨胀难以倒出药渣，加入药材之前需要将较大饮片适当捣碎处理；最终加入提取得到的挥发油，应在药液温度冷至常温后加入，并需要增溶处理后加入。

（3）白芷进行渗漉可以避免香豆素成分受热损失。操作中，白芷需要粉粹成粗粉，粉碎不可过细，并注意装筒松紧度要适中，不可过紧也不可过松。渗漉时需要控制适当流速，一般为 1~3ml/min。润湿时，加入药材量的 1~2 倍溶媒。最终渗漉液用量一般为药材量的 8 倍。

（4）药液的醇沉处理中，需要将药液温度降至室温，乙醇的加入方式采用多次醇沉、慢加快搅，如此有助于提高醇沉效果。醇沉静置一般需要 24 小时，密闭冷藏有利于药液中各物质溶解度降低而沉淀析出。

（二）质量检查

1. **性状**　本品应为棕褐色的液体；气微香，味苦、辛，微甜。

2. **pH**　照 pH 测定法（通则 0631），应为 4.0~6.0。

3. **相对密度**　比重瓶法（通则 0601）测定，应不低于 1.07。

4. **装量**

（1）单剂量灌装的合剂　取供试品 5 支，将内容物分别倒入经标化的量入式量筒内，在室温下检视，每支装量与标示装量相比较，少于标示装量的不得多于 1 支，并不得少于标示装量的 95%，应符合规定。

（2）多剂量灌装的合剂　照最低装量检查法（通则 0942）检查，应符合规定。

5. **微生物限度**　除另有规定外，照非无菌产品微生物限度检查：微生物计数法（通则 1105）和控制菌检查法（通则 1106）及非无菌药品微生物限度标准（通则 1107）检查，应符合规定。

思考题

1. 中药合剂（口服液）处方中含挥发油的药材饮片应如何处理？最终采用什么方式将挥发油加入口服液？

2. 简述渗漉法的优点与适用性。

3. 中药合剂（口服液）制备的工艺流程都有哪几步？

4. 中药合剂（口服液）配液中一般需要加入哪些附加剂？

5. 浅谈如何解决中药合剂（口服液）的沉淀问题。

题库

Experiment 2 Preparation of Chinese Herbal Mixture (oral liquid)

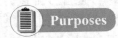 **Purposes**

1. To master the preparation methods, key operations and precautions of traditional Chinese medicine mixture (oral liquid).

2. To be familiar with the routine quality requirements and inspection methods of traditional Chinese medicine mixture (oral liquid).

3. To understand filling equipment for traditional Chinese medicine mixtures (oral liquid).

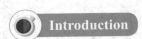 **Introduction**

1. Traditional Chinese medicine mixture refers to the oral liquid preparation, prepared by extracting the traditional Chinese medicine pieces with water or other solvent, by the appropriate method. The single dose of packaging is called "oral liquid". Traditional Chinese medicine mixture (oral liquid) is an improved and developed traditional Chinese medicine dosage form based on traditional decoction.

2. Characteristics. Traditional Chinese medicine mixture (oral liquid) inherits the advantages of absorptio n and rapid effect of traditional Chinese medicine decoction, meanwhile, it does not need to be boiled before use, and it is convenient to use. As a concentrated product of decoction, the dosage is reduced. However, during the storage of mixture, a small amount of volatile precipitation often occurs. Mixture relative to the presence of decoction can not be added or subtracted with symptoms; Production process is relatively complex, production equipment, high requirements for technological conditions.

3. The preparation process of traditional Chinese medicine mixture (oral liquid) is as follows (Figure 2-1):

(1) Pretreatment of Chinese medicinal materials　Cleanly select→washing→ moistening → cutting → drying → clean the pieces.

(2) Extraction　Generally, suitable extraction methods are selected according to the solubility of the main chemical components contained in the decoction pieces of medicinal materials. The commonly used solvents are water and ethanol. Due to the polarity of water, most of them use decoction method; Ingredients are generally first extracted by double extraction, that is, the aromatic volatile ingredients are first extracted by steam distillation, and the residue is then decocted with other medicinal materials in the prescription.

(3) Concentration　Concentration is the evaporation of the solvent to increase the concentration of the solution, which is the dehydration operation. The concentration of the extract of traditional Chinese

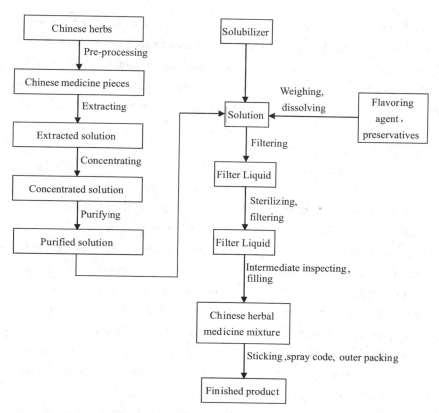

Figure 2-1   The preparation process of traditional Chinese medicine mixture coral liquid

medicine mixture (oral liquid) will affect the effect of purification. The appropriate concentration method and conditions should be selected according to the thermal stability of the components of the prescription drugs. Generally, the amount of prescription extract is often large, which brings inconvenience to the next purification operation. For example, using the water alcohol method, if the concentration of the medicine solution is too thin, the amount of alcohol needed to reach a certain alcohol concentration is large, which also causes troubles in alcohol precipitation, filtration, ethanol recovery and other processes. Generally concentrated to a relative density of about 1.0 (50~60℃) or 1~2g/ml equivalent to the original medicinal materials.

(4) Purification   The usual purification methods are high-speed centrifugation, water and alcohol, alcohol and water, adsorption and clarification. The selection of purification method and its parameters (such as alcohol content, amount of clarifying agent and centrifugal speed, etc.) should be based on the content of the drug components.

(5) Reconcentration   After extraction and purification, the prescription Chinese medicine still needs to be concentrated properly. If the extract of traditional Chinese medicine refined by alcohol precipitation contains ethanol, water and other solvents, the ethanol in the alcohol precipitation supernatant needs to be fully recovered by decompression concentration first, and then part of the solvent water is removed by atmospheric pressure evaporation concentration, so as to meet the requirements of mixture preparation and molding. The concentration level is generally 10~20ml per dose.

(6) Mixing liquid   In order to make the Chinese medicine mixture has a good taste and stability, should be in a clean, germ-free environment operation, can add the appropriate flavor correction agent, antiseptic, pH regulator, solvent and antioxidant. Taste masking agent. If the mixture USES sucrose as a flavor correction agent, the sucrose content is generally not higher than 20% (g/ml). The preservatives

sorbic acid and sodium benzoate shall not exceed 0.3%, and the dosage of hydroxybenzoate shall not exceed 0.05%. The varieties and dosage of preservatives added shall comply with the relevant provisions of the national standards, and shall not affect the stability of the mixture finished products, and shall avoid interference to the inspection, when necessary, an appropriate amount of ethanol can be added.

(7) Filtration　The filtration of prescription decoction extracts is mostly filtered by centrifuge or plate-and-frame filter, and the purified liquid and the prepared liquid are treated by plate-and-frame filter and tube-type centrifuge by coarse filter and fine filter (0.22μm) respectively.

(8) Filling and sterilization　The prepared liquid should be filled in sterile clean and dry suitable container with negative pressure mixture filling machine or perfusion oral liquid filling line as soon as possible. According to the material of the filling bottle, the appropriate sterilization method is selected. The glass bottle terminal is sterilized, and the methods of boiling sterilization, hot pressing sterilization and high temperature instantaneous sterilization are adopted after filling. The plastic bottles are sterilized first with fine filtrate and then filled, and most of them are sterilized intermittently at low temperature. After sterilization, the bottles are filled after the temperature of the liquid medicine drops.

4. The percolation method is a dynamic leaching method, which can maintain a good concentration gradient during the extraction process, high extraction efficiency, easy operation, room temperature operation, and does not destroy the heat-sensitive components. Extraction of medicinal herbs. The process of the single infiltration method is: crushing of the medicinal material→wetting→filling the tube→exhausting→dipping →percolating→leachate.

5. Quality requirements. It showld be clarified, no mildew, rancidity, foreign matter, discoloration, generation of gas or other deterioration during the storage period, nonetheless a small amount of easily dispersed sediment may be allowed. General should check relative density, pH value, etc. Single-dose and multi-dose filling mixture shall be inspected for filling capacity and microbial limit, and shall meet the requirements.

 Equipments and Materials

1. Equipments　Furnace (or induction cooker, infrared heating furnace), 1000ml electric heating jacket, soaking tube, water bath, 100ml round bottom flask, volatile oil separator, condensation tube, (circulating water or electronic) vacuum pump, Buchner funnel, alcohol meter, (1 in 10,000) electronic balances, electronic balances, pH meters, pycnometers, mills (or pounding tanks), 1.5ml plastic centrifuge tubes, etc.

2. Materials　Notopterygium Rhizoma, Ledebouriellae Radix, Atractylodis Rhizoma, Asari Herba, Chuanxiong Rhizoma, Angelicae Dahuricae, Scutellariae Radix, Glycyrrhizae Radix, Rehmanniae Radix, medical alcohol, polysorbate 80, sorbate sucrose, distilled water, distilled water.

 Experimental Procedures

（Ⅰ）Preparation of Jiuwei Qianghuo Oral Liquid

【Formula】

Notopterygium Rhizoma　30g	Ledebouriellae Radix　30g
Atractylodis Rhizoma　30g	Asari Herba　10g
Chuanxiong Rhizoma　30g	Angelicae Dahuricae　20g

Scutellariae Radix   20g   Glycyrrhizae Radix   20g

Rehmanniae Radix   20g

【Preparation】 Above nine kinds of Chinese medicines, Angelicae Dahuricae are crushed into coarse powder, and the percolation method under the terms of the flow-through extracts and extracts (General rule 0189), using 8 times the amount of 70% ethanol as the solvent, soaking for 24 hours, and percolation method, collect mash and reserve. Notopterygium Rhizoma,Ledebouriellae Radix,Atractylodis Rhizoma,Herba Asari Rhizoma Chuanxiong were extracted the volatile oil by adding 6 times water,and collect the distilled aqueous solution in another device. The dregs and the remaining Scutellariae Radix and other three Chinese medicines are decoated twice with (10, 8 times) water for 1h at a time. Combine the decoction and filter. The filtrate is combined with the above aqueous solution and concentrated to about 180ml. The supernatant and the mash were combined, ethanol was recovered, and concentrated to a clear paste having a relative density of 1.10 to 1.20 (70°C), diluted by water to 160ml, and put it aside. 20g of sucrose was made into a single syrup by the hot-melt method and set aside. Add volatile oil to 0.4ml of polysorbate 80, add a small amount of medicinal solution, mix well, then add medicinal solution, single syrup and 0.2g of sorbic acid, mix well and add water to 200ml. Mix, aliquot, and sterilize.

Experiment flow chart (Figure 2–2):

【Characters】 This product should be a brown liquid.

【Functions and Indications】 Disperse the wind and dehydrate the table, disperse cold and dehumidify. It is used for colds caused by exogenous wind chills and dampness. The symptoms include chills, fever, no sweat, heavy head pain and limb pain.

【Usage and dosage】 Oral administration. 20ml once, 2~3 times a day.

【Considerations】

(1) In the prescription of Jiuwei Qianghuo Oral Liquid, there are more volatile components in the five herbal pieces of Notopterygium Rhizoma, Ledebouriellae Radix, Atractylodis Rhizoma, Asari Herba and chuanxiong Rhizoma. Modern research shows that the volatile oils contained in these medicinal materials are its effective ingredients, so the double extraction method is adopted here.

(2) In view of the prescription, the five kinds of medicinal herbal medicines, such as Notopterygium Rhizoma, Ledebouriellae Radix, Atractylodis Rhizoma, Asari Herba and chuanxiong Rhizoma, contain less than 1 proportion of volatile oil. Therefore, a light oil volatile oil extractor must be used. In order to improve the yield of volatile oil, and prevent the expansion of the medicine after extracting the volatile oil from being difficult to pour out the medicine residue.The larger decoction pieces are appropriately mashed and treated; the volatile oil obtained after the extraction is finally added, the temperature of the liquid medicine is cooled to normal temperature, and it is added after the solubilization treatment.

(3) Angelicae Dahuricae percolation can prevent the loss of coumarin components from heat. During operation of Angelicae Dahuricae percolation, Angelicae Dahuricae powder into coarse powder, crushing should not be too fine, and pay attention to the barrel tightness should be moderate, the tube tightness should be moderate, not too tight and not too loose, the percolation needs to control the appropriate flow rate, generally 1~3ml/min. When wetting, adding 1~2 times the amount of medicinal materials solvent, modern research the final amount of percolation liquid is generally 8 times the amount of medicinal materials.

(4) In the alcohol precipitation treatment of the medicinal solution, the temperature of the medicinal solution needs to be lowered to room temperature. The method of adding ethanol uses multiple alcohol

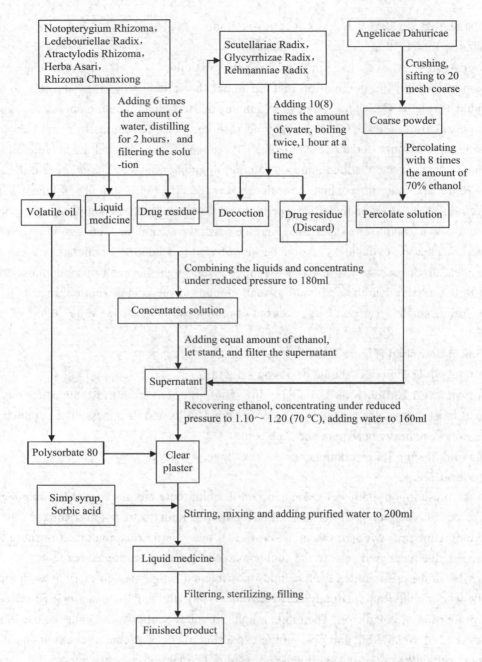

Figure 2-2 The preparation flow chart of Jiuwei Qianghuo Oral Liquid

precipitations and slow and fast stirring, which helps to improve the alcohol precipitation effect. Alcohol sedimentation usually requires 24 hours, and sealed refrigeration will help reduce the solubility of various substances in the drug solution and precipitate.

（Ⅱ）Quality Inspection

1. Characters The character of this product should be tan liquid; gas micro fragrance, bitter, spicy, slightly sweet.

2. pH According to the pH measurement method (General rule 0631), it should be 4.0~6.0.

3. Relative density Specific gravity bottle method (General rule 0601) determination, should not be less than 1.07.

4. Volume

Single-dose Filling Mixture Take 5 samples, pour the contents into the marked-up gauge tube separately, and inspect them at room temperature. The quantity of each sample shall not be more than 1 less than the marked quantity and not less than 95% of the marked quantity.

Multi-dose Filling Mixture Inspection shall be in accordance with the minimum quantity inspection act (General rule 0942).

5. Microbial limits Unless otherwise specified, inspection of microbial limits for non-sterile products: microbial counting method (General rule 1105) and control bacteria inspection method (General rule 1106) and non-sterile drug microbial limit standard (General rule 1107) shall comply with the regulations.

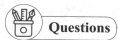 **Questions**

1. How to deal with the pieces of volatile oil in the prescription of traditional Chinese medicine mixture (oral liquid)? What is the final way to add the volatile oil into the oral liquid?

2. Please briefly describe the advantages and applicability of percolation.

3. What is the technological process of preparation of traditional Chinese medicine mixture (oral liquid)?

4. What additional agent does Chinese traditional medicine oral liquid need to add commonly in mix liquid?

5. Talking about how to solve Chinese traditional medicine mixture (oral liquid) precipitation problem.

实验三　药酒和糖浆剂的制备

 实验目的

1．**掌握**　一般药酒及糖浆剂的制备方法及其操作要点。
2．**熟悉**　浸渍法、渗漉法原理及操作过程。
3．**了解**　影响浸出效率的因素。

实验提要

1．药酒系指将药物置于 75% 乙醇或白酒中浸泡而成。为提高浸出效率，可以采取适度粉碎药物、提高浸出温度、掌握适宜的浸出时间、扩大浓度差等方法。

2．糖浆剂系指含有药物、药材提取物或芳香物质的口服浓蔗糖水溶液。供口服使用。含糖量应不低于 45%（g/ml）。蔗糖及芳香剂等能掩盖药物的不良气味，改善口味，尤其受儿童欢迎。糖浆剂易被微生物污染，低浓度的糖浆剂中应添加防腐剂。常用的防腐剂中苯甲酸和山梨酸的用量不得超过 0.3%，对羟基苯甲酸酯类的用量不得超过 0.05%。防腐剂对微生物的抑制作用有一定的选择性，故常使用混合防腐剂以增强防腐效能。

3．浸渍法。浸渍法是将药材与适量的溶剂放入密闭容器中，浸渍一定时间后进行固液分离，将浸渍液添加溶剂到全量的提取方法。该方法为低温提取，不加热或加热温度低；药材与溶剂处于相对静止的状态，一定时间后固体与液体之间有效成分交换达到动态平衡，有效溶出量不再增加；浸渍法所用溶剂增多，药渣吸液可能造成有效成分损失。浸渍法适用于没有细胞结构、新鲜的药材、吸液膨胀率大、含热敏成分的药材及低浓度制剂，不适用于贵重药材的提取和高浓度制剂的制备。

4．渗漉法。渗漉法系将药材粗粉置渗漉器内，溶剂连续从渗漉器上部加入，渗漉液不断从下部流出，从而浸出药材中有效成分的方法，属于动态低温浸渍法。该法有效成分提取率高，提取彻底。而且渗滤液可以做下次渗漉的渗漉用液，药液的浓度不断增加。适合于贵重药、有效成分含量低的药材、热敏性成分的提取及高浓度制剂的制备。但不适用于新鲜易膨胀的药材、无细胞结构的药材。渗漉法根据操作方法的不同，可分为单渗漉法、重渗漉法、加压渗漉法、逆流渗漉法。

实验器材

1．**仪器**　烧杯、玻璃棒、量筒、天平、滤纸、渗漉筒、纱布、小瓷片、表面皿等。
2．**试药**　蕲蛇（去头）、羌活、红花、防风、五加皮、当归、秦艽、牡丹皮、白芍、浙贝母、玄参、麦冬、生地、甘草、薄荷油、白酒、蔗糖、单糖浆等。

实验操作步骤

（一）蕲蛇药酒的制备

【处方】

蕲蛇（去头）	12g
羌活	6g
红花	9g
防风	3g
五加皮	6g
当归	6g
秦艽	6g

【制法】

（1）粉碎、润湿　蕲蛇粉碎成粗粉，其余防风等6味混合粉碎成粗粉，与上述粗粉混合均匀，置烧杯中，加入白酒适量（约35ml），拌匀，浸润0.5小时，使其充分膨胀。

（2）装筒、浸渍　装入底部填有脱脂棉的渗漉筒中，层层轻压，装好后于药面上覆盖滤纸1张，并压小瓷片数块，打开出液口，自上部加白酒并保持液面高于粉柱上平面，流出液不夹带气泡时，关闭出液口，加白酒使其高出药面1~2cm，密闭，浸渍48小时。

（3）渗漉　以白酒为溶剂，按渗漉法调节流速为1~3ml/min，缓缓渗漉，收集渗漉液约900ml。

（4）配制　向渗漉液中加入蔗糖10g，搅拌溶解后，滤过，加入适量白酒，制成1000ml，即得。

实验流程图如图3-1所示。

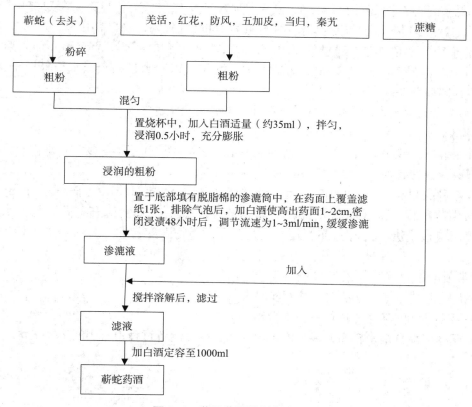

图 3-1　蕲蛇药酒的制备流程图

【性状】本品为棕黄色的澄清液体；气香，味苦、微甜。允许底部有少量轻摇即散的沉淀。

【注意事项】药物粉碎也不宜过粗，否则，会导致渗漉筒堵塞。同时，渗漉筒底部的脱脂棉必须处于疏松状态。白酒应高于药面 1~2cm，同时流速不宜太快。

（二）养阴清肺糖浆的制备

【处方】

白芍	6g
浙贝母	6g
玄参	10g
牡丹皮	6g
麦冬	9g
生地黄	15g
甘草	3g
薄荷油	0.1g
单糖浆 54ml（相当于总量约30%）	共制成 180ml

【制法】

1. 提取　取白芍、浙贝母、玄参、麦冬、生地黄、甘草六味药共 49g，加水没过药面（约 50ml）浸泡 0.5 小时后，直火加热，煮沸后 25 分钟加入牡丹皮，继续煎煮至 1 小时，以双层纱布滤过；再加水没过药面，煎煮 45 分钟，滤过，合并两次滤液。浓缩至每 1ml 相当于原生药 1g。放冷，加乙醇使含醇量为 60%。置冰箱中静置过夜，滤过，滤液回收乙醇至无味后，以煮沸过的蒸馏水稀释至180ml。

2. 配制

（1）单糖浆的制备　取蒸馏水 45ml，煮沸，加入蔗糖 85g，搅匀，溶解后继续加热至 100℃，用脱脂棉滤过，自滤器上补加适量热蒸馏水，使全量为 100ml，搅匀，放冷待用。

（2）含药糖浆的配制　以适量的 95% 乙醇约 10ml，将 0.1g 薄荷油溶解并加入溶液中，混匀加入相当于总体积 30%（约 54ml）的单糖浆，混匀，以煮沸过的蒸馏水稀释至全量，即得。

实验流程图如图 3-2 所示。

【性状】本品为棕褐色的液体；气香，味甜、微苦，有清凉感。

【质量检查】

（1）外观性状　除另有规定外，糖浆剂应澄清。在贮存期间不得有发霉、酸败、产生气体或其他变质现象，允许有少量摇之易散的沉淀。

（2）含糖量的测定　一般采用手持糖量计进行测定，含蔗糖量应不低于 45%（g/ml）。

（3）微生物限度　除另有规定外，照非无菌产品微生物限度检查：微生物计数法（通则 1105）和控制菌检查法（通则 1106）及非无菌药品微生物限度标准（通则 1107）检查，应符合规定。

【注意事项】

（1）乙醇为易燃物品，实验时应注意实验安全。

（2）滤液必须无醇味才能进行下一步操作。

（3）由于糖浆剂含糖量较高，极易滋生微生物，故在制备过程中所用的蒸馏水均应煮沸。

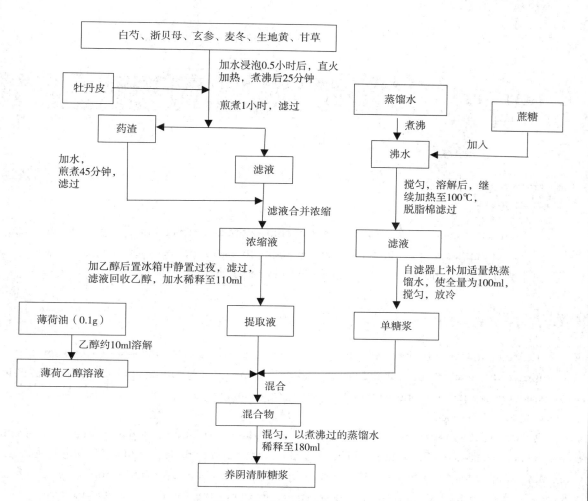

图 3-2　养阴清肺糖浆的制备流程图

🖊️ **思考题**

1. 渗漉法与浸渍法有哪些异同点？

2. 糖浆剂制备过程中有哪些注意事项？单糖浆与糖浆剂的区别有哪些？

3. 糖浆剂测定含醇量的意义是什么？

4. 煎煮过程中操作要点有哪些？

Experiment 3　Preparation of Medicinal Wine and Syrup

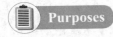

Purposes

1. To master the preparation methods and operation points of general medicine liquor and syrup.
2. To be familiar with the principle and operation process of impregnation and percolation.
3. To understand the factors affecting the leaching efficiency.

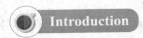

Introduction

1. Medicinal wine refers to the medicine which is soaked in 75% alcohol or white spirit. In order to improve the leaching efficiency, we can take some methods, such as appropriate pulverization of drugs, increasing the leaching temperature, mastering the appropriate leaching time, and enlarging the concentration difference.

2. Syrup refers to the oral concentrated sucrose aqueous solution containing drugs, herbal extracts or aromatic substances. For oral use. The sugar content shall be not less than 45% (g/ml). Sucrose and aromatics can mask the bad smell of drugs and improve taste, especially popular with children. Syrup is easy to be polluted by microorganism. Preservative should be added to syrup with low concentration. The amount of benzoic acid, sorbic acid and p-hydroxybenzoic acid esters in common preservatives shall not exceed 0.3% and 0.05%, respectively. Preservatives have certain selectivity to the inhibition of microorganisms, so mixed preservatives are often used to enhance the anti-corrosion effect.

3. The method of maceration put the medicinal materials and a certain amount of solvent into a closed container. After maceration for a certain period of time, the solid-liquid separation is carried out, and the maceration solution is added to the full amount of solvent. The method is low temperature extraction, no heating or low heating temperature; the medicine and solvent are in a relatively static state, after a certain period of time, the exchange of effective components between the solid and the liquid reaches a dynamic balance, and the effective dissolution does not increase any more; the increase of solvents used in the immersion method may cause the loss of effective components. The impregnation method is suitable for medicine without cell structure, fresh medicine, high swelling rate of liquid absorption, medicine with thermosensitive components and low concentration preparation, not suitable for extraction of precious medicine and preparation of high concentration preparation.

4. The infiltration method is a method of placing the coarse powder of medicinal materials in an infiltrator, the solvent is continuously added from the upper part of the infiltrator, and the infiltrating solution continuously flows out from the lower part, thereby leaching the effective ingredients in the medicinal material, which belongs to the dynamic low-temperature impregnation method. This method

24

has a high extraction rate of active ingredients and complete extraction. In addition, the leachate can be used as an infiltration solution for the next infiltration, and the concentration of the medicinal solution is continuously increasing. It is suitable for the extraction of precious medicines, medicinal materials with low active ingredient content, heat-sensitive ingredients, and the preparation of high-concentration preparations. But it is not suitable for fresh and swellable medicinal materials and medicinal materials without cell structure. Infiltration method can be divided into single infiltration method, heavy infiltration method, pressure infiltration method and countercurrent infiltration method according to different operation methods.

 Equipments and Materials

1. Equipments　Beakers, glass rods, measuring cylinders, balances, filter paper, infiltration canisters, gauze, small porcelain plates, watch glasses, etc.

2. Materials　Agkistrodon (without head), Notopterygium root, safflower, Sileris Radix, Acanthopanax Radicis Cortex, Angelicae Sinensis Radix, Gentiana, Moutan Cortex, Paeoniae Radix, Bulb of Thunberg Fritillary, Scrophulariae Radix, Ophiopogon japonicus, dried rehmannia root, liquorice, peppermint oil, white spirit, sucrose, single syrup, etc.

 Experimental Procedures

（Ⅰ）Preparation of Agkistrodon Wine

【Formula】

Prescription: Agkistrodon (without head)　12g

Notopterygium root　6g

Safflower　9g

Sileris Radix　3g

Acanthopanax Radicis Cortex　6g

Angelicae Sinensis Radix　6g

Gentiana　6g

【Preparation】

(1) Crush and moisten the Agkistrodon into coarse powder, mix and crush the other 6 flavors of radix sileris into coarse powder, mix with the above coarse powder, put it in a beaker, add a proper amount of liquor (about 35ml), mix well, soak the dense group for 0.5h, and make it fully expand.

(2) The bottom of the cartridge and immersion container is filled with absorbent cotton in the percolation cartridge, which is pressed gently layer by layer. After loading, the filter paper is covered on the drug surface, and several pieces of small porcelain pieces are pressed. The liquid outlet is opened. Liquor is added from the upper part and the liquid level is kept higher than the upper plane of the powder column. When there is no bubble in the liquid outlet, the liquid outlet is closed. Liquor is added to make it 1 to 2cm higher than the drug surface, sealed and soaked for 48h.

(3) For percolation, the liquor is used as the solvent, and the flow rate is adjusted from 1 to 3ml per minute according to the percolation method. The percolation fluid is collected about 900ml

(4) Preparation, add 10g sucrose into the percolate, stir and dissolve it, filter it, add some white spirit, to 1000ml.

Experimental flow chart (Figure 3-1):

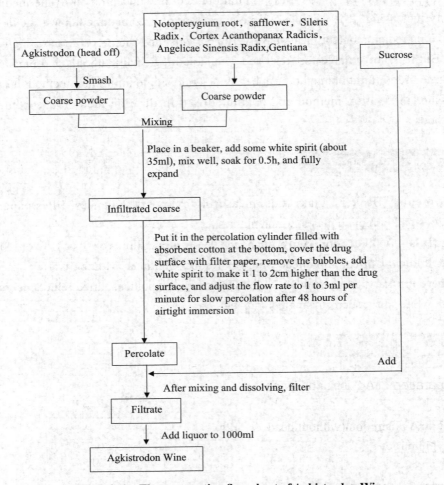

Figure 3-1　　The preparation flow chart of Agkistrodon Wine

【Characters】This product is the brown clear liquid, fragrant, bitter and slightly sweet. A small amount of precipitate is allowed at the bottom.

【Considerations】Drug should not be crushed too thickly, otherwise, the percolation cylinder will be blocked. At the same time, the absorbent cotton at the bottom of the percolation drum must be in a loose state. The liquor should be 1 ~ 2cm higher than the drug surface, and the flow rate should not be too fast.

(Ⅱ) Preparation of Syrup for Yangyin Qingfei

【Formula】

Paeonia Lactiflora	6g
Fritillaria thunbergii	6g
Scrophulariae Radix	10g
Cortex Moutan	6g
Dwarf lilyturf	9g
Rehmanniae Radix	15g
Licorice	3g
Peppermint oil	0.1g
Single syrup 54ml(Equivalent to about 30% of the total)	180ml in total

26

【Preparation】

1. Extrac Take 49g of six kinds of herbs, that are Paeonia Lactiflora, fritillaria thunbergii, Scrophulariae Radix, dwarf lilyturf, Rehmanniae Radix, and Licorice; soak it in water (about 50ml) for 0.5h, heat it by direct fire, add in the Cortex Moutan after boiling for 25min, continue to boil it for 1h, and filter it with double gauze; add water to set up medicine noodles, decoct for 45min, filter it and combine the filtrate twice. Concentrate to 1g per 1ml. Cool down and add ethanol to make the alcohol content 60%. Put it in the refrigerator overnight, filter it, recover ethanol from the filtrate until it is tasteless, and dilute it to 180ml with boiling distilled water.

2. Preparation

(1) Preparation of single syrup: Take 45ml distilled water, boil it, add 85g sucrose, stir well, after dissolving, continue heating to 100℃, filter with absorbent cotton, add appropriate amount of hot distilled water to the self-filter, make the total amount to 100ml, stir well, cool and set aside.

(2) Preparation of medical syrup: Dissolve 0.1g peppermint oil in an appropriate amount of 95% ethanol about 10ml, add it into the solution, mix it with single syrup equivalent to 30% of the total volume (about 54ml), mix it well, dilute it to the full amount with boiled distilled water.

Experimental flow chart (Figure 3–2):

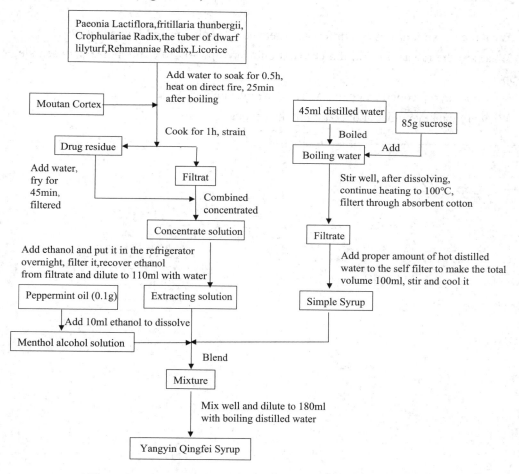

Figure 3–2　The preparation flow chart of Yangyin Qingfei Syrup

【Characters】This product is a brown liquid; it is fragrant, sweet, slightly bitter and cool.

【Quality Inspection】

(1) Appearance Unless otherwise specified, syrup shall be clarified. During storage, there shall be no

mildew, rancidity, gas generation or other deterioration, and a small amount of precipitate which is easy to disperse by shaking is allowed.

(2) Determination of sugar content　The sugar content is generally measured by hand-held sugar meter, and the sugar content shall not be less than 45% (g/ml).

(3) Microbial limit　Unless otherwise specified, the microbial limit of non sterile products shall be inspected according to the microbial count method (General rule 1105), control bacteria inspection method (General rule 1106) and the microbial limit standard of non sterile drugs (General rule 1107), which shall meet the requirements.

【Considerations】

(1) Ethanol is a kind of inflammable substance, so we should pay attention to the safety of the experiment.

(2) The filtrate must be alcohol free before the next operation.

(3) Due to the high sugar content of syrup, microorganisms are easily to grow, distilled water used in the preparation process should be boiled.

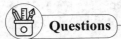 **Questions**

1. What are the similarities and differences between percolation and impregnation?

2. What are the precautions in the preparation of syrup? And the difference between single syrup and syrup?

3. Why does syrup contain alcohol? What is the meaning?

4. What are the key points of operation in the decocting process?

实验四 煎膏剂的制备

实验目的

1. 掌握 煎膏剂的制备方法。

2. 熟悉 含糖量、相对密度的测定方法。

3. 了解 煎膏剂的质量检查方法。

实验提要

1. 煎膏剂系指饮片用水煎煮，取煎煮液浓缩，加炼蜜或糖（或转化糖）制成的半流体制剂。

2. 煎膏剂的制备工艺流程：煎煮 → 浓缩 → 收膏 → 分装 → 成品。

（1）煎煮 药材一般以煎煮法浸提。药材饮片加水煎煮 2~3 次，每次 2~3 小时，合并煎液，备用。

（2）浓缩 将浸提液浓缩至规定的相对密度，即得清膏。

（3）炼糖 取蔗糖加入糖量 1/2 的水及 0.1% 的酒石酸，加热溶解保持微沸，至糖液呈金黄色，转化率达 40%~50%。

（4）收膏 清膏中加入规定量的炼糖或炼蜜，不断搅拌，继续加热熬炼至规定的标准即可。除另有规定外，加炼糖和炼蜜的量一般不超过清膏量的 3 倍。收膏时的相对密度一般在 1.40 左右。

（5）分装与贮藏 煎膏剂应分装在洁净干燥灭菌的大口容器中，待充分冷却后加盖密闭。煎膏剂应贮藏于阴凉干燥处。

3. 煎膏剂的特点：浓度高、体积小、稳定性好、便于服用，主要用于滋补，又称膏滋，同时具有缓和的治疗作用，多用于慢性疾病。但热敏药物、挥发性药物不易制成膏滋。

实验器材

1. **仪器** 烧杯、电热炉、糖量计、韦氏比重瓶。

2. **试药** 益母草、红糖、酒石酸、蒸馏水。

实验操作步骤

（一）益母草膏的制备

【处方】

益母草	50g
红糖	15g
0.1% 酒石酸	适量

【制法】将益母草置于烧杯中，加水高于药材3~4cm，煎煮两次，每次0.5小时，合并煎液，滤过，浓缩至相对密度1.21~1.25（80~85℃）的清膏。称取红糖，加糖量1/2的水及0.1%的酒石酸，直火加热熬炼，不断搅拌至呈金黄色时，加入上述清膏，继续浓缩至规定的相对密度，即得。

实验流程图如图4-1所示。

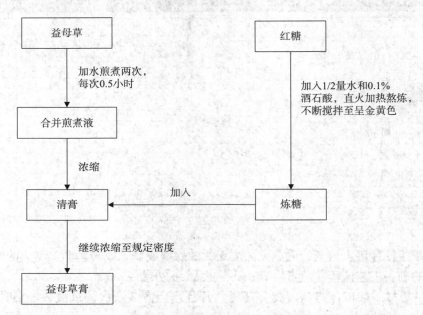

图4-1　益母草膏的制备流程图

【性状】本品为棕黑色稠厚的半流体，气微，味苦、甜。

【功能与主治】清热解毒、祛瘀止痛、活血调经等。

【用法与用量】每日三次，每次10ml，直接服用或加水服用。

【注意事项】儿童禁用，肾、肝功能不全者慎用。不宜与肾上腺素、异丙肾上腺素、阿托品同用。

（二）益母草膏的质量检查

1. **性状**　煎膏剂应无焦臭、异味，无糖的结晶析出。

2. **含糖量**　一般用糖量计测定制剂的含糖量。

3. **相对密度的测定**　除另有规定外，照相对密度测定法（通则0601）测定。取本品10g，加水20ml稀释后，相对密度应为1.10~1.12。

4. **不溶物**　取供试品5g，加热水200ml，搅拌使溶化，放置3分钟后观察，不得有焦屑等异物。

5. **微生物限度**　照非无菌产品微生物限度检查：微生物计数法（通则1105）和控制菌检查（通则1106）及非无菌药品微生物限度标准（通则1107）检查，应符合规定。

题库

思考题

1. 煎膏剂的制备过程应注意哪些问题？如何防止煎膏出现"反砂"现象？

2. 按传统方法收膏的标准有哪些？

Experiment 4　Preparation of Concentracted Decoctions

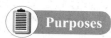

Purposes

1. To master the preparation method of concentracted decoctions.
2. To be familiar with the determination of sugar content and relative density.
3. To understand the quality inspection method of concentracted decoctions.

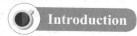

Introduction

1. Concentracted decoctions are semi-fluid preparation prepared by decocting the crude drug in water, concentrating the decoction to a smaller volume an adding previously-refined honey or sugar (or invert-sugar) to form the final product.

2. The preparation process of concentracted decoctions: decocting → concentrating → collecting → packaging → products.

(1) Decoction　Herbs are generally extracted by decoction. Add water into the decoction pieces of medicinal materials and decoct 2~3 times, each time for 2~3h. Then combine the decoctions.

(2) Concentration　Filter the above decoctions, and concentrated to a thin extract with specified relative density.

(3) Sugar refining　The sucrose is added with 1/2 of water and 0.1% tartaric acid, then the solution is heated and kept slightly boiling until the sugar solution turns golden yellow with a conversion rate of 40% ~ 50%.

(4) Collection　Add specified amount of refined sugar into the thin extract, stir constantly, and continue to heat refining to the specified standard. Unless otherwise specified, the amount of refined sugar should not exceed 3 times the amount of refined sugar. The relative density of the concentracted decoctions is generally about 1.40.

(5) Package and storage　Concentracted decoctions should be packaged in a clean, dry and sterilized large-mouth container, and sealed after being cooled sufficiently. The concentracted decoctions should be stored in a cool and dry place.

3. Characteristics of concentracted decoctions: high concentration, small volume, good stability and easy to take. It is mainly used for tonic, also known as "Gaozi". At the same time, the concentracted decoctions has a mild therapeutic effect and mostly used for chronic diseases. But thermosensitive drugs and volatile drugs are not easy to make into concentracted decoctions.

Equipments and Materials

1. Equipments　Beaker, electric heater, sugar meter, wechsler pycnometer.

2. Materials　Leonuri Herba, brown sugar, tartaric acid, distilled water.

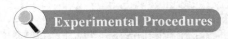 **Experimental Procedures**

（Ⅰ）Preparation of Yimucao Gao

【Formula】

Leonuri Herba	50g
Brown sugar	15g
0.1% tartaric acid	q.s.

【Preparation】Leonuri Herba are placed into a beaker, add water into the beaker until it is 3~4cm above the crude drugs. Decoct the crude drug twice, 0.5h each time. Combined the decoctions, filtered, and concentrate to a thin extract with relative density of 1.21~1.25 (80~85℃). Weigh the brown sugar, add water (equal to 1/2 amount of sugar) and 0.1% tartaric acid. Melt by direct-flame heating under continuous stirring until its color becomes golden yellow. Add the above extract, mix well, and continuously concentrate to the specified relative density.

Experiment flow chart (Figure 4-1):

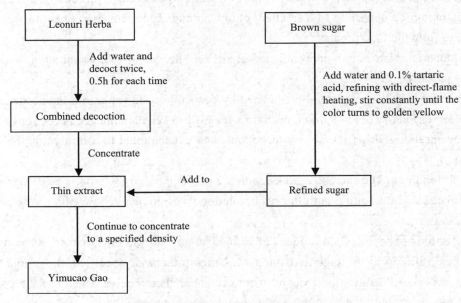

Fiugure 4-1　The preparation of Yimucao Gao

【Characters】This product is a brownish-black and thick semifluid with slight odour, tastes bitter and sweet.

【Functions and Indications】Clearing heat and detoxification, removing blood stasis and relieving pain, activating blood circulation and regulating menstruation.

【Usage and Dosage】10ml every time, three times a day, for oral administration either directly or with water.

【Considerations】Children are not allowed to use. Kidney and liver with care. Leonuri decoction paste should not be used with adrenaline, isoproterenol or atropine.

（Ⅱ）Quality inspection of Yimucao Gao

1. Characteristics　The product should be no smell, odour, sugar-free crystallization.

2. The sugar content　The sugar content of the concentrated decoction is determined by a sugar meter.

3. Relative density　Unless otherwise specified, the relative density of the concentrated decoction is determined according to the specific gravity bottle method (General rule 0601). After 10g of the product is diluted with 20ml of water, the relative density should be 1.10~1.12.

4. Insoluble substance　Take 5g of the test product and place it in a breaker, and into 200ml of hot water, stir to dissolve, leave for 3min and observe. There should be no foreign bodies such as coke chips.

5. Microbial limit　Test for non-sterile products: microbial count test (General rule 1105), control bacteria test (General rule 1106), and microbial limit test for non-sterile drugs (General rule 1107) shall be conducted in accordance with the requirements.

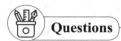 **Questions**

1. What problems should be paid attention to in the preparation of concentracted decoctions? How to prevent the concentracted decoctions from appearing "Fansha" phenomenon?

2. What are the traditional methods of collecting the thick extract?

PPT

实验五　液体制剂的制备

实验目的

1. **掌握**　不同类型液体制剂的制备方法、常用附加剂、关键操作和注意事项。
2. **熟悉**　混悬剂中附加剂的应用。
3. **了解**　液体制剂的质量检查方法。

实验提要

　　液体制剂是指药物分散在适宜介质中制成的液体形态的制剂。按分散系统可将液体制剂分为：均相液体制剂和非均相液体制剂。

　　1. 溶液剂是指药物以分子或离子状态（小于 1nm）分散于介质中制成的内服或外用的液体形态的制剂。常用的溶剂有水、乙醇、甘油、丙二醇等。溶液型液体制剂外观均匀、澄明。属于溶液剂的有溶液剂、芳香水剂、甘油剂、醑剂和糖浆剂等，溶液剂通常采用溶解法、稀释法和化学反应法制备，一般制备过程为：称量→溶解→混合→过滤→加溶媒至全量→检查→包装→成品。

　　2. 乳剂是指互不相溶的两种液体混合，其中一种液体以液滴状态分散于另一种液体中形成的非均匀相液体分散体系，一般粒径在 0.1~100μm。乳剂可以分为 O/W 型或 W/O 型，是一种热力学和动力学不稳定的分散体系，在制备过程中需要通过一定的机械力作用进行分散，同时加入乳化剂。乳化剂可以降低界面张力，提高乳化膜的稳定性，常用的乳化剂有各种表面活性剂、阿拉伯胶、西黄蓍胶等。乳剂的制备方法有油中乳化剂法（干胶法）、水中乳化法（湿胶法）、新生皂法及两相交替加入法。小量制备乳剂可采用干胶法，先将胶粉与油混合，应注意容器的干燥，研磨均匀后，加少量水相充分研磨均匀形成初乳后，稀释得乳剂。

　　3. 混悬剂是指难溶性固体药物以微粒状态分散于分散介质中所形成的非均匀的液体制剂，可供口服、局部外用和注射。为了提高混悬剂的稳定性，常需在混悬剂中加入稳定剂，如助悬剂、润湿剂、絮凝剂和反絮凝剂。混悬剂的制备方法有分散法（如研磨粉碎）和凝聚法（如化学反应和微粒结晶）。研磨粉碎一般制备过程为：取药物 1 份加液体 0.4~0.6 份研磨，同时加入润湿剂，研细后，加分散介质稀释以及添加助悬剂和絮凝剂或反絮凝剂。

实验器材

　　1. **仪器**　天平、量筒、研钵、具塞玻璃瓶、滤纸、玻璃漏斗、烧杯、蒸发皿、水浴锅、玻璃棒、试管夹、七号筛。
　　2. **试药**　薄荷油、滑石粉、甲酚、豆油、氢氧化钠、软皂、松节油、樟脑、生大黄、沉降硫、液化酚、甘油、CMC-Na、聚山梨酯 80、蒸馏水。

（一）薄荷水的制备

【处方】

薄荷油	0.2ml
滑石粉	1.5g
蒸馏水	加至 100ml

【制法】 称取滑石粉，置于干燥研钵中，加入薄荷油，充分搅匀。量取适量的蒸馏水，分次加入研钵中，先加入少量，研匀后再逐渐加入其余的蒸馏水，每次都要研匀。最后将混合液移入具塞玻璃瓶中，并用蒸馏水将钵体中的滑石粉冲洗入玻璃瓶，加入蒸馏水，加盖，振摇 10 分钟。滤过至澄明，再由滤器上添加适量蒸馏水，使成 100ml，即得。

实验流程图如图 5-1 所示。

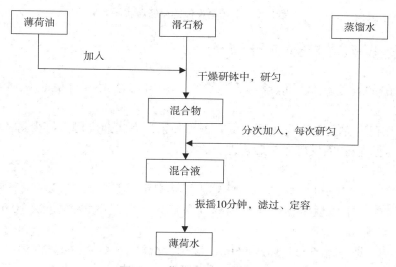

图 5-1　薄荷水的制备流程图

【性状】 本品为澄清水溶液，具有薄荷香气。

【功能与主治】 芳香矫味与驱风药。用于胃肠胀气，亦可用作药剂的溶剂。

【注意事项】

（1）本品为薄荷油的饱和水溶液，处方用量为溶解量的 4 倍，配制时不能完全溶解。

（2）滑石粉为分散剂，可增加薄荷油的分散度，加速其溶解，并可以吸附剩余的薄荷油，以利于溶液的澄清。但所用的滑石粉不宜过细，以免滤液混浊。若第一次滤过后仍不澄清，可再回滤，直至形成澄明溶液。

（3）制备时，应将薄荷油与滑石粉充分研磨至分散均匀。

（二）甲酚皂溶液的制备

【处方】

甲酚	25ml
植物油	9g
氢氧化钠	1.35g
水	加至 50ml

【制法】

（1）称取氢氧化钠 1.35g，加入 5ml 蒸馏水，加热使之溶解。

（2）称取植物油 9g，水浴加热至 80℃。

（3）向（2）中加入氢氧化钠溶液使发生皂化反应，用玻璃棒不断搅拌，搅拌过程中加入少量乙醇（制品全量的 5.5%），以加速皂化过程，搅拌至出现肥皂样为止。

（4）加入 25ml 甲酚溶液，搅拌，蒸发皿不离开水浴锅，待皂化液澄清，移走，放冷。

（5）放冷后，加蒸馏水至 50ml，搅拌使之混匀，即得。

实验流程图如图 5-2 所示。

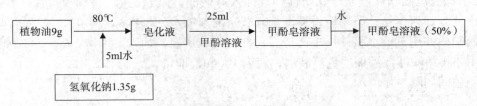

图 5-2　甲酚皂溶液的制备流程图

【性状】 甲酚皂溶液为微黄色的透明溶液。

【注意事项】

（1）甲酚与酚的性质相似，但杀菌力较酚强，较高浓度时，对皮肤有刺激性，操作时应注意。

（2）该法皂化程度完全与否与成品质量有密切关系，皂化速度可因加少量乙醇（约占制品全量的 5.5%）而加速反应，而反应完全后再加热除醇。

【质量检查】

（1）碱度　取本品 1.0ml，加中性乙醇（对酚酞指示液显中性）20ml 稀释后，加酚酞指示液 1.0ml，如显红色，用硫酸滴定液（0.05mol/L）滴定，消耗硫酸滴定液（0.05mol/L）不得过 1.0ml。

（2）未皂化物　取本品 5ml，加水 95ml，混匀，溶液应澄清；如显混浊，与对照液（取标准硫酸钾溶液 6ml，加水 80ml 与稀盐酸 1ml，用比色用氯化钴液和浓焦糖液调色，色调与供试品溶液近似后，加 25% 氯化钡溶液 3ml，并加水至 100ml，摇匀，放置 10 分钟）比较，不得更浓。

（三）松节油搽剂的制备

【处方】

软皂	7.5g
樟脑	5.0g
松节油	65.0ml
蒸馏水	加至 100ml

【制法】 称取软皂与樟脑至研钵内，研磨至液化，缓缓加入松节油，研磨均匀后，分数次注入储有蒸馏水 25ml 的具塞玻璃瓶中，边加边用力振摇，乳化完全后，加蒸馏水至 100ml，摇匀即得。

实验流程图如图 5-3 所示。

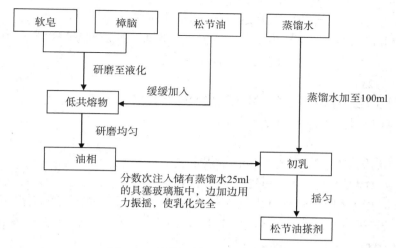

图 5-3　松节油搽剂的制备流程图

【性状】本品为乳白色至微黄色乳状液体，有特臭。

【功能与主治】刺激皮肤，使局部充血、发红。用于扭伤、肌肉痛、关节痛、神经痛等症。

【注意事项】本品系干胶法制备。软皂与樟脑研匀后，松节油应分次缓缓加入，沿同一方向大力研匀。使用的研钵应干燥。

【质量检查】

（1）乙醇中不溶物　取本品 1ml，加 95% 乙醇 7ml，振摇使溶解，溶液应澄清。

（2）相对密度测定　照通则 0601 检查，应不低于 0.87。

（3）其他　应符合通则 0117（搽剂）有关各项规定。

（四）颠倒散洗剂的制备

【处方】

生大黄	3.75g
沉降硫	3.75g
液化酚	0.5ml
甘油	5.0ml
CMC-Na	0.25g
聚山梨酯 80	2.5g
蒸馏水	加至 50ml

【制法】生大黄、沉降硫研细过七号筛，将细粉置于研钵中，加液化酚、甘油、CMC-Na、聚山梨酯 80 研匀后再加液研磨，加水至 50ml 即得。

实验流程图如图 5-4 所示。

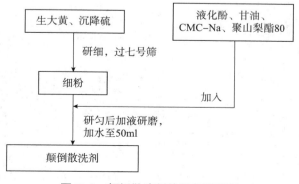

图 5-4　颠倒散洗剂的制备流程图

【性状】本品为黄棕色混悬液，久置后分层，但振摇后易分散。

【功能与主治】软化表皮，杀寄生虫。用于疥疮、体癣、痤疮和脂溢性皮炎等。

【用法与用量】用前摇匀，外搽患处，每日 3~4 次。

【注意事项】

（1）沉降硫疏水性极强，加甘油、聚山梨酯 80 做润湿剂。

（2）加液研磨时应分次加入蒸馏水，研匀。

【质量检查】

（1）装量　照通则（0942）检查，应符合规定。

（2）无菌检查　照通则（1101）检查，应符合规定。

（3）细菌内毒素或热原　除另有规定外，照通则（1143）或热原检查法通则（1142）检查，每 1ml 中含细菌内毒素的量应小于 0.50 EU 内毒素，应符合规定。不能进行细菌内毒素检查的冲洗剂应符合热原检查法的规定。

 思考题

1. 滑石粉在制备薄荷水中，能否用其他物质代替？

2. 薄荷水除了用上述的分散溶解法制备外，能否用其他方法制备？

3. 制备甲酚皂溶液的原理是什么？

4. 试写出甲酚皂溶液制备过程中，有哪些植物油可取代豆油？

5. 松节油搽剂不稳定易分层，其原因是什么？

6. 颠倒散洗剂中各组成物质起何作用？硫黄为何选用沉降硫？

题库

Experiment 5 | Preparation of Liquid Dosage Forms

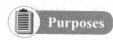 **Purposes**

1. To master the preparation methods, common additives, key operations and precautions of different types of liquid preparations.

2. To be familiar with the usage of the suspending agent in suspensions.

3. To understand the quality inspection method for the liquid preparations.

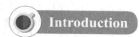 **Introduction**

Liquid dosage forms are preparations containing medicaments dispersed in a suitable meduim. The liquid formulation is classified into homogeneous and heterogeneous liquid dosage forms based on the dispersion system.

1. Solution preparations are liquid preparations containing medicaments dissolved in a suitable solvent to form a solution for internal or external use, the drugs are dispersed in dispersion solvent as molecular or ionic state (proton diameter less than 1nm), Water, alcohol, glycerol and propylene glycol are the most frequently used solvent. A liquid preparation in solution should be uniformity and clarity. They are usually prepared by the methods of solution, dilution, and chemical reaction method. General preparation procedures are as follows: weighting, dissolution, mixing, filtering, adding solvent to the whole, checking, packaging, and labeling.

2. The emulsion is defined as two immiscible liquids, one of which is finely subdivided and uniformly distributed as droplets throughout the other to form a non-homogeneous dispersion system, the general diameter is among 0.1μm to 100μm. The types of emulsions include oil in water (O/W) type and water in oil (W/O) type. The methods for emulsion preparation include emulsifier in oil method (dry glue method), emulsifier in water method (wet glue method), nascent soap method and alternate addition method. A small amount of emulsion can be prepared by dry glue method, first, mix the rubber powder and oil phase in a dried container, after grinding evenly, add a small amount of water phase, then continuous grinding to form colostrum, diluted with water phase.

3. Suspensions are liquid preparation containing insoluble solid medicaments dispersed in liquid dispersing medium. The suspension is used in pharmacy in many different dosage forms and can be taken orally, applied topically or injected. In order to improve the stability of suspensions, stabilizers usually used in preparation of suspensions, such as suspending agents, wetting agents, flocculation agents or deflocculation agents. The preparation methods of suspension include dispersing method (such as grinding) and coacervation method (such as micro-particle crystallization and chemical reaction). The general process of grinding with liquid to prepare suspensions are taken one copy medication and add liquid 0.4~0.6 copies, then grinding while adding an appropriate amount of wetting agent, after grinding,

39

diluted with dispersion and added suspending agent, flocculation agent or deflocculation agent.

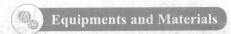 **Equipments and Materials**

1. Equipments   Balance, measuring cylinder, mortar, glass bottle with stopper, filter paper, glass funnel, beaker, evaporation dish, water bath, glass rod, test tube clip, sieve (No.7).

2. Materials   Peppermint oil, talcum powder, cresol, soybean oil, sodium hydroxide, soft soap, turpentine oil, camphor, raw rhubarb, precipitated sulfur, liquefied phenol, glycerin, sodium salt of carboxy methyl cellulose (CMC-Na), polysorbate 80, distilled water.

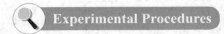 **Experimental Procedures**

（Ⅰ）Preparation of Peppermint Water

【Formula】

Peppermint oil	0.2ml
Talcum powder	1.5g
Distilled water	Add to 100ml

【Preparation】Weigh 1.5g of talcum powder, put it in a dried mortar, add peppermint oil, and stir well. Measure an appropriate amount of distilled water, add it to the mortar in stages, add a small amount first, after grinding, then add the remaining distilled water gradually and grind each time. Then, transfer the mixture into a glass bottle with a plug and rinse the talcum powder in the bowl into the glass bottle with distilled water. Cover with plug, shake for 10 min, filter to clear, and add an appropriate amount of distilled water to the filter to 100ml, obtain.

Experiment flow chart (Figure 5-1):

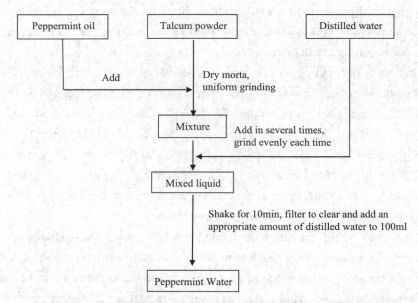

Figure 5-1   The praparation procedure of Peppermint Water

【Characters】This product is a clear aqueous solution with a mint aroma.

【Functions and Indications】Fragrance and dispelling wind medicine. Used for flatulence and as a solvent for medicaments.

【 Considerations 】

(1) This product is a saturated aqueous solution of peppermint oil. The prescription dosage is 4 times of the dissolved amount. It cannot be completely dissolved when prepared.

(2) Talcum powder is a dispersant, which can increase the dispersion of peppermint oil, accelerate its dissolution, and can adsorb the remaining peppermint oil to facilitate the clarification of the solution. However, the talcum powder used should not be too fine, so as not to make the filtrate cloudy. If it does not clear after the first filtration, it can be filtered back until a clear solution is formed.

(3) During preparation, the peppermint oil and talcum powder should be fully ground until they are uniformly dispersed.

(II) Preparation of Saponated Cresol Solution

【 Formula 】

Cresol	25ml
Soybean oil	9g
Sodium hydroxide	1.35g
Water	Add to 50ml

【 Preparation 】

(1) The sodium hydroxide was roughly weighed as 1.35g in a beaker, and 5ml distilled water was added and heated to dissolve it.

(2) 9g soybean oil was roughly weighed by evaporation dish and heated to 80℃ in a water bath.

(3) Adding sodium hydroxide solution to the evaporation dish (containing soybean oil) to cause saponification reaction, stirring continuously with a glass rod, adding a small amount of ethanol (5.5% of the total amount of the product) in the stirring process to add the saponification process and stirring until the soap sample appears.

(4) Measure the 25ml cresol solution in the measuring cylinder, pour it into the evaporation dish (containing saponification liquid), stir with a glass rod, do not leave the water bath, wait for the saponification solution to be clarified, remove and let cool.

(5) Pour into 50ml beaker after cooling, add distilled water to 50ml, stir and mix well.

Experiment flow chart (Figure 5-2):

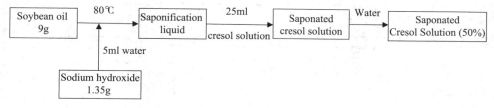

Figure 5-2　The praparation proceclure of Saponated Cresol Solution

【 Characters 】 This product is a yellowish transparent solution.

【 Considerations 】

(1) The properties of cresol and phenol are similar, but the bactericidal power is stronger than phenol. When the concentration is higher, it is irritating to the skin, so the operation should be careful.

(2) Whether the saponification degree of the method is complete or not is closely related to the quality of the finished product. The saponification rate can be accelerated by adding a small amount of ethanol (about 5.5% of the total product), and the reaction is complete and then heated to remove the alcohol.

【Quality Inspection 】

(1) Alkalinity   Take 1.0ml of this product, add neutral ethanol (neutral to phenolphthalein indicator) 20ml dilution, add phenolphthalein indicator 1.0ml, if red, titrate with sulfuric acid titration solution (0.05mol/L), consumption sulfuric acid titration solution (0.05mol/L) must not pass 1.0ml.

(2) Unsaponifiable matter   Take 5ml of this product, add water 95ml, mix well, and the solution should be clarified; if it is turbid, it should not be thicker than the control solution (6ml of standard potassium sulfate solution, adding water 80ml and dilute hydrochloric acid 1ml, coloring with colorimetric solution of cobalt chloride and concentrated caramel, hue similar to the test solution, adding 25% barium chloride solution 3ml, adding water to 100ml, shaking well, and leaving for 10 minutes).

（Ⅲ） Preparation of Turpentine Oil Liniment

【Formula 】

Soft soap	7.5g
Camphor	5.0g
Turpentine oil	65.0ml
Distilled water	Added to 100ml

【Preparation 】Put the soft soap and camphor in the mortar, grind it to liquefy, slowly add turpentine oil, grind it evenly, and then pour it into a glass bottle with a stopper containing 25ml of distilled water. Shake vigorously while adding. After emulsification is complete, add distilled water to 100ml and shake well.

Experiment flow chart (Figure 5–3):

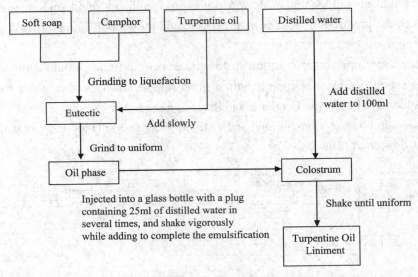

Figure 5–3   The preparation procedure of Turpentine Oil Liniment

【Characters 】This product is a milky white to slightly yellow milky liquid with a specific odor.

【Function and Indications 】Stimulate the skin, make local congestion and redness. For sprains, muscle pain, arthralgia, neuralgia, etc.

【Considerations 】This emulsion is prepared by the emulsifier in oil method. After the soft soap and camphor are homogenized, turpentine oil should be added slowly in stages and vigorously homogenized in the same direction. The mortar used should be dry.

【Quality Inspection 】

(1) Insoluble matter in ethanol   Take 1ml of this product, add 7ml of 95% ethanol, shake to

dissolve, the solution should be clear.

(2) Determination of relative density   Checked according to the General rule 0601 It should be no less than 0.87.

(3) Others   It shall comply with the relevant provisions of General rule 117 (Tincture).

（Ⅳ）Preparation of Diandaosan Lotion

【Formula】

Raw rhubarb	3.75g
Precipitated sulfur	3.75g
Liquefied phenol	0.5ml
Glycerine	5.0ml
CMC–Na	0.25g
Polysorbate 80	2.5g
Distilled water	Add to 50ml

【Preparation】Raw rhubarb and precipitated sulfur are crushed into the fine powder and passed through No. 7 sieve. The fine powder is put into a mortar, evenly grind with liquefied phenol, glycerin, CMC-Na and polysorbate 80. Then add the liquid and continue grinding, and finally add water to 50ml.

Experiment flow chart (Figure 5–4):

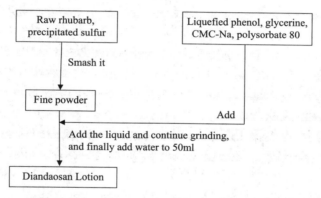

Figure 5–4   The preparation of Diandaosan Lotion

【Characters】It is a yellow-brown suspension, layering occurs over time, but easy to disperse after shaking.

【Functions and Indications】Soften the skin and kill the parasites. Used for scabies, ringworm, acne, seborrheic dermatitis and etc.

【Usage and Dosage】Shake well before use, rub the affected part outside, 3~4 times a day.

【Considerations】

(1) Precipitated sulfur has a strong hydrophobicity, with glycerin, polysorbate as a lubricant.

(2) Add distilled water and grind separately.

【Quality Inspection】

(1) Loading capacity   The inspection examining minimum loading capacity (General rule 0942) should comply with the provisions.

(2) Sterility test   According to the aseptic examination method (General rule 1101) and should comply with the regulations.

(3) Bacterial endotoxin or pyrogen   Unless otherwise specified, bacterial endotoxin test (General rule 1143) or pyrogen test (General rule 1142) should be performed in accordance with the requirements. The amount of bacterial endotoxin in 1ml should be less than 0.50 EU endotoxin. Lotions that cannot be tested for bacterial endotoxin should comply with the pyrogen test.

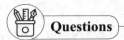 **Questions**

1. Whether or not talcum powder can be replaced by other substances in the preparation of peppermint water?

2. In addition to the above method, can peppermint water be prepared by other methods?

3. What is the principle of preparing saponated cresol solution?

4. Give the preparation process of saponated cresol solution, which vegetable oils can replace soybean oil in the preparation of saponated cresol solution?

5. Diandaosan lotion is unstable and easy to layer. What is the reason?

6. What is the effect of the constituent substances in Diandaosan Lotion? Why precipitated sulfur?

实验六　注射剂的制备

PPT

实验目的

1. **掌握**　无菌与灭菌制剂生产工艺中的关键操作。
2. **熟悉**　注射剂生产的（手工）工艺过程和操作要点。
3. **了解**　注射剂成品质量检查标准和方法及其影响因素。

实验提要

1. 注射剂系指用药物制成的供注入体内的无菌溶液、乳状液和混悬液，以及供临用前配成溶液或混悬液的无菌粉末。

2. 注射剂起效迅速，剂量准确，特别是可用作急救危重患者用的静脉滴注的输液。由于注射剂直接注入体内，吸收快，所以对生产过程和质量控制，都要求极其严格。

3. 注射剂的灭菌方法，应根据灭菌的药物及其制剂的稳定性进行选择。

4. 按分散系统不同，中药注射剂可分为溶液型、混悬液型、乳浊液型和注射用无菌粉末等。按注射方式不同，中药注射剂可分为静脉注射剂、肌内注射剂、穴位注射剂或局部病灶注射剂等。

5. 注射剂的质量要求为无菌、无热原、澄明度合格、使用安全、无毒性和刺激性、稳定性合格，即在贮存期内稳定有效。注射液的 pH 一般控制在 4~9 范围内，大剂量静脉注射或滴注的输液，应调节渗透压与血浆渗透压相等或接近。凡在水溶液中不稳定的药物，常制成注射用灭菌粉末（即粉针剂），制备方法有冷冻干燥法、灭菌溶剂结晶法、喷雾干燥法等，以保证注射剂在贮存期内稳定、安全、有效。

6. 对于有效成分清楚的中药注射剂，应选择适宜的溶媒和方法，提取有效成分，再按注射剂的工艺流程进行制备。中药注射液常用的提取纯化方法如下。

（1）溶媒处理法　水提醇沉、醇提水沉。
（2）蒸馏法　适用于含挥发性成分药材的提取方法。
（3）双提法　蒸馏法和水提法结合的方法。
（4）超滤法　用于分子分离的膜滤过法。

实验器材

1. **仪器**　不锈钢杯、电炉、石棉网、天平、称量纸、玻璃棒、抽滤瓶、真空泵、注射器、烧杯（250ml）、牛角勺、量筒、G4 垂熔玻璃漏斗、安瓿、澄明度检测仪、微孔滤膜、砂芯过滤装置、pH 试纸、熔封机、镊子、蒸发皿、电炉、水浴锅、三角烧瓶等。
2. **试药**　丹参、亚硫酸氢钠、注射用水。

医药大学堂
www.yiyaodxt.com

💬 实验操作步骤

（一）空安瓿的前处理

1. **洗涤**　将每支安瓿灌满滤过的蒸馏水，以 100℃、30 分钟热处理，甩水（热甩一次），再如上法灌水、甩水，反复两次（冷甩两次）。

2. **干燥**　将洗好的安瓿置烘箱内用 120℃ 温度干燥 2 小时，备用。

（二）容器处理

配制用的一切容器，均需清洗保证洁净，避免引入杂质及热原。

（三）滤器处理

1. **垂熔玻璃漏斗**　先用水反冲，除去上次药液留下的杂质，沥干后用洗液浸泡处理，用水冲尽，最后用注射用水过滤至滤出的水 pH 检查不显酸性，澄明度检查合格为止。

2. **微孔滤膜**　常用的是由醋酸、硝酸纤维素混合酯组成的微孔滤膜，使用前将其浸泡于注射用水中 1 小时，煮沸 5 分钟，如此反复 3 次，使滤膜中纤维充分膨胀，增加滤膜韧性。使用时用镊子取出滤膜且使毛面向上，平放在膜滤器的支撑网上，注意滤膜不要被皱摺，装好后应完整无缝隙，无泄漏现象，用注射用水过滤，滤出水澄明度合格，即可将滤器盖好备用。

（四）注射液（丹参注射液）的配制

【处方】

丹参	200g
亚硫酸氢钠	0.3g
注射用水	加至 100ml

【制法】

（1）**制备浓缩液**　称取丹参饮片 200g，加蒸馏水浸泡 30 分钟，煎煮两次，第一次加 8 倍量水煎煮 40 分钟，第二次加 5 倍量水煎煮 30 分钟，用双层纱布分别滤过，合并滤液，浓缩至约 100ml（每毫升相当于原药材 2.0g）。

（2）**纯化**

醇处理：于浓缩液中加无水乙醇使含醇量达 75%，静置冷藏 40 小时以上，双层滤纸抽滤，滤液回收乙醇，并浓缩至约 20ml，再加无水乙醇使含醇量达 85%，静置冷藏 40 小时以上，同法滤过，滤液回收乙醇，浓缩至约 15ml。

水处理：取上述浓缩液加 10 倍量蒸馏水，搅匀，静置冷藏 24 小时，双层滤纸抽滤，滤液浓缩至约 100ml，放冷，再用同法滤过 1 次，用 20% NaOH 调 pH 6.8~7.0。

活性炭处理：在上述浓缩液中加入 0.2% 活性炭，煮沸 20 分钟，稍冷后抽滤。水浴浓缩至25ml。

（3）**配液**　取上述滤液，加入亚硫酸氢钠 0.3g，溶解后，加注射用水至 100ml，先粗滤，再用 G4 垂熔漏斗抽滤。

（4）**灌封**　在无菌室内，用手工灌注器灌装，每支 2.0ml，封口。

（5）**灭菌**　煮沸灭菌，100℃，30 分钟。

（6）**检漏**　剔除漏气安瓿。

（7）**灯检**　剔除有白点、色点、纤维、玻璃屑及其他异物的成品安瓿。

（8）**印字**　擦净安瓿，用手工印上品名、规格、批号等。

（9）**包装**　将安瓿装入衬有瓦楞纸的空盒内，盒面印上标签。

实验流程图如图 6-1 所示。

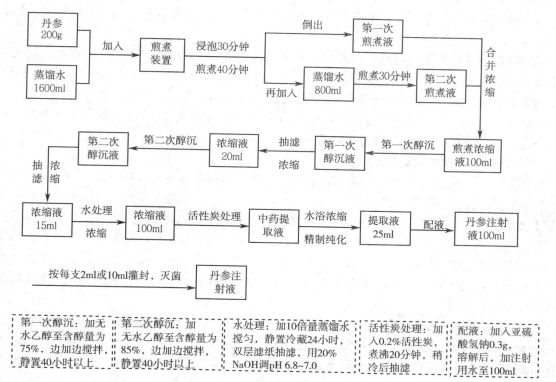

图 6-1　丹参注射液的配制流程图

【性状】本品为红棕色澄明液体。

【功能与主治】活血化瘀，用于冠状动脉供血不足，心肌缺氧所引起的心绞痛、心肌梗死等。

【用法与用量】肌注，一次 2.0ml，每日 1~2 次。

【注意事项】

（1）本品为丹参经提取制成的灭菌、棕色的澄明水溶液，每 1ml 相当于丹参 2g。

（2）丹参注射液是中药制剂，保存不当可能影响产品质量。使用前必须对光检查，如发现药液出现混浊、沉淀、变色、漏气或瓶身细微破裂者，均不能使用。

（3）丹参注射液在生产与贮藏期间均应符合下列有关规定：①应无异臭、无酸败味；除另有规定外，色泽不得深于黄色 6 号标准比色液，在 10℃ 时应保持澄明。②碘值为 79~128；皂化值为 185~200；酸值不大于 0.56。其他溶剂必须安全无害，用量应不影响疗效。

（4）配制注射剂时，可按药物的性质加入适宜的附加剂。附加剂如为抑菌剂时，用量应能抑制注射液内微生物的生长。常用的抑菌剂（g/ml）为 0.5% 苯酚、0.3% 甲酚、0.5% 三氯叔丁醇等。加有抑菌剂的注射液，仍应用适宜的方法灭菌。注射量超过 5ml 的注射液，添加的抑菌剂必须特别慎重选择。供静脉或椎管注射用的注射液，均不得添加抑菌剂。

除另有规定外，容器应符合国家标准中有关药用玻璃容器的规定。容器胶塞应符合有关规定。

（5）配制注射液时，灌注的药液必须澄明，容器应洁净干燥后使用。配制注射用油溶液时，应先将精制的油在 150℃ 干热灭菌 1~2 小时，并放冷至适宜的温度。供直接分装成注射用无菌粉末的原料药应无菌，凡用冷冻干燥法者，其药液应无菌，灌装时装量差异应控制在 ±4% 以内。

（6）注射剂在配制过程中，应严密防止变质与污染微生物、热原等。已调配的药液应在当日内完成灌封、灭菌，如不能在当日内完成，必须将药液在不变质与不易繁殖微生物的条件下保存；供静脉及椎管注射用的注射剂，更应严格控制。

（7）药液在不变质与不易繁殖微生物的条件下保存；供静脉及椎管注射用的注射剂，更应严格控制。

（8）接触空气易变质的药物，在灌装过程中，容器内应排除空气，填充二氧化碳或氮气等气体后熔封。

（9）熔封或严封后，可根据药物的性质选用适宜的方法灭菌，必须保证成品无菌。

（10）熔封的注射剂在灭菌时或灭菌后，应采用减压法或其他适宜的方法进行容器检漏。

（11）注射剂应按规定的条件避光贮藏。

（五）注射剂的常规质量检查

1. **装量**　注射液及注射用浓溶液照下述方法检查，应符合规定。

检查法：供试品标示装量不大于2ml者，取供试品5支（瓶）；2ml以上至50ml者，取供试品3支（瓶）。开启时注意避免损失，将内容物分别用相应体积的干燥注射器及注射针头抽尽，然后缓慢连续地注入经标化的量入式量筒内（量筒的大小应使待测体积至少占其额定体积的40%，不排尽针头中的液体），在室温下检视。测定油溶液、乳状液或混悬液时，应先加温（如有必要）摇匀，再用干燥注射器及注射针头抽尽后，同前法操作，放冷，检视。每支（瓶）的装量均不得少于其标示量。

2. **装量差异**　除另有规定外，注射用无菌粉末按照下述方法进行检查，应符合规定。

检查法：取供试品5瓶（支），除去标签、铝盖，容器外壁用乙醇擦净，干燥，开启时注意避免玻璃屑等异物落入容器内，分别迅速精密称定；容器为玻璃瓶的注射用无菌粉末，首先小心开启内塞，使容器内外气压平衡，盖紧后精密称定。称定后倾出内容物，容器用水或乙醇清洗，在适宜条件下干燥后，再分别精密称定每一容器的重量，求出每瓶的装量与平均装量。每瓶（支）装量与平均装量比较（如有标示装量，则与标示装量相比较），应符合下列规定（表6-1），如有不符合规定，应另取10瓶（支）复试，应符合规定。

表6-1　注射剂装量差异限度

平均装量或标示装量	装量差异限度
0.05g 及 0.05g 以下	±15%
0.05g 以上至 0.15g	±10%
0.15 以上至 0.50g	±7%
0.50g 以上	±5%

凡规定检查含量均匀度的注射用无菌粉末，一般不再进行装量差异检查。

3. **渗透压摩尔浓度**　除另有规定外，静脉输液及椎管注射用注射液按各种品项下的规定，照渗透压摩尔浓度测定法（通则0632）检查，应符合要求。

4. **可见异物**　除另有规定外，照可见异物检查法（通则0904）检查，应符合规定。

5. **不溶性颗粒**　除另有规定外，用于静脉注射、静脉滴注、鞘内注射、椎管内注射的溶液型注射液、注射用无菌粉末及注射用浓溶液照不溶性颗粒检查法（通则0903）检查，应符合规定。

6. **中药注射剂相关物质**　按各品种项下规定、照注射剂有关物质检查法（通则2400）检查，应符合有关规定。

7. **重金属及有害元素残留量**　除另有规定外，中药注射剂按照铅、镉、砷、汞、铜测定法（通则2321）测定，按各品种项下每天最大使用量计算，铅不得超过12μg，镉不得超过3μg，砷不得超过6μg，汞不得超过2μg，铜不得超过150μg。

8. **无菌** 照无菌检查法（通则 1101）检查，应符合规定。

9. **细菌内毒素或热原** 除另有规定外，静脉用注射剂按各品种项下的规定，照细菌内毒素检查法（通则 1143）或热原检查法（通则 1142）检查，应符合规定。

思考题

1. 中药注射剂目前存在的主要问题有哪些，应如何应对？

2. 注射剂中常用的附加剂种类和品种有哪些？注射剂中附加剂选用的原则是什么？

3. 中药注射用原液的制备方法还有哪些？"水醇法"制备中药注射剂的依据是什么？

4. 中药注射剂和化药注射液的制备有何异同？

Experiment 6 Preparation of Injections

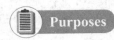

Purposes

1. To master the concept of sterility through experiments and master the key operations in the production process of sterility and sterilization preparations.

2. To be familiar with the (manual) process and key points of operation of injection production.

3. To understand the quality inspection standards and methods of injection products and their influencing factors.

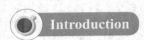

Introduction

1. Injections refers to sterile solutions, emulsions, and suspensions made of drugs for injecting into the body, and sterile powders that are formulated as solutions or suspensions before use.

2. Quick effect and accurate dosage are its prominent characters, and consequently intravenous drips of infusions are usually used for emergency treatment. Because the injection is directly injected into the body and rapidly absorbed, the extremely strict requirements are demanded on its production process and quality control.

3. The sterilization method of injection should be selected according to the stability of sterilized drugs and their formulation.

4. According to the dispersion system, traditional Chinese medicine injections (TCMJ) can be classified into solution, suspension, emulsion and sterile powder for injection. According to the injecting ways, TCMJ can be sorted into intravenous injection, intramuscular injection, acupoint injection or local focus injection, etc.

5. The quality requirements for injection include sterility, free of pyrogens, clarity, safety, nontoxicity, tissues tolerance and stability. The pH of injection is generally controlled in the range of 4 to 9. For large volume intravenous fluids, the osmotic pressure should be adjusted to equal or close to the plasma osmotic pressure.

6. The active ingredients in the preparations should be extracted with appropriate solvent and effective methods, and injection prepared according to process. Common use extraction and purification methods are as follows:

(1) Treatment by solvent: including water extraction and alcohol precipitation method, and alcohol extraction and water precipitation method.

(2) Distillation method: a method applicable to the herbs containing volatile ingredients.

(3) Double extraction: the combination of distillation and water extraction.

(4) Ultra-filtration: a membrane filtration method for molecular separation.

Equipments and Materials

1. Equipments Stainless steel cup, electric furnaces, asbestos mesh, balances, weighing paper, glass rods, suction filter bottles, vacuum pumps, syringes, beakers (250ml),horn spoons, measuring tubes, G4 siloed glass funnel, ampoule, luminosity detectors, hmicroporous filter membrane, sand core filtering device, pH test paper, melting machines, tweezers, evaporation furnaces, electric furnace, water bath pot, triangular flask, etc.

2. Materials Salviae Miltiorrhizae Radix, sodium bisulfite, water for injection.

Experimental Procedures

（Ⅰ）Disposal of Empty Ampoules

1. Washing Fill each ampoule with filtered distilled water, heat treat at 100°C for 30 minutes, splash water (throw off the hot water, once), then fill water and swing water as above, repeat twice (throw off cool water, twice).

2. Drying Put the washed ampoules into an oven at 120°C for drying 2 hours,reserved.

（Ⅱ）Container Handling

All containers used for preparation must be cleaned, cleanliness and free-introduction of impurities and progeny.

（Ⅲ）Filter Treatment

1. Falling glass funnel Backflushing with water to remove the previous impurities, draining, soaking with lotion, flushing with water, and finally filtering with injection water until the filtered-water is not acidic and the clarity is qualified.

2. Microporous filter membrane The common one is a kind of microporous filter membrane composed of acetic acid and nitrocellulose mixed ester, which is soaked in injection water for 1.0 hour and boiled for 5.0 minutes before use. Repeat this process 3 times to fully expand the fibers and increase the toughness. When using the filter membrane, take it outwith tweezers, face up the rough surface, lay it flat on the support net of the membrane filter. Please pay attention to the filter membrane that does not to be wrinkled, the finishedinstallment should be complete,seamless, no leakage.It should be filtered with injection water until the clarity is qualified. The whole filter installmentshould be covered while preserved.

（Ⅳ）Preparation of Injection (Danshen Injection)

【Formula】

Salviae Miltiorrhizae Radix	200g
Sodium bisulfite	0.3g
Water for injection	Add to 100ml

【Preparation】

(1) Weigh Salviae Miltiorrhizae Radix 200g, soak it in distilled water for 30 min, and decoct it twice: 8 times water and 40 min for the first time, 5 times water and 30 min for the second time. Filtering it with double gauze respectively, mixing filtrates, and concentrating it to 100ml or so (2.0g original medicinal materials per 1ml solution).

(2) Purification

Treat with alcohol: Adding ethanol into the concentrated solution to make the alcohol content reach

75%, standing and refrigerating for over 40h, filtering with double-layer filter paper. Recovering ethanol, concentrating to about 20ml, then adding ethanol to reach 85%, standing and refrigerating for more than 40h, filtering as the same method, recovering ethanol, and concentrating to about 15ml.

Treat with water: Add 10 times of distilled water to the above-concentrated solution, stir evenly, let stand and refrigerate for 24h, filter with double-layer filter paper, concentrate the filtrate to about 100ml, cool, filter again as the same method, and adjust its pH to 6.8 ~ 7.0 with 20% NaOH.

Treat with activated carbon: 0.2% activated carbon is added to the upper liquid; the solution is boiled for 20 min, and filtered after slightly cooling. It was concentrated to 25ml by a water bath.

(3) Solution preparation　Take out the above filtrate, add 0.3g sodium bisulfite, dissolute it, add water for injection to make the solution reach 100ml. The solution was first filtered roughly and then filtered with a G4 vertical melting funnel.

(4) Filling　In a sterile room, fill with a manual perfusion device, each 2.0ml, sealed.

(5) Sterilization　Boiling sterilization, 100℃, 30min.

(6) Leak detection　Remove leaky ampoules.

(7) Light inspection　Remove the finished ampoule with white spots, color spots, fibers, glass shavings, and other foreign matter.

(8) Printing　Wipe the ampoule clean and manually print the name, specification, batch number, etc.

(9) Packaging　Put ampoules into empty boxes lined with corrugated paper, and label the boxes.

Experiment flow chart (Figure 6–1):

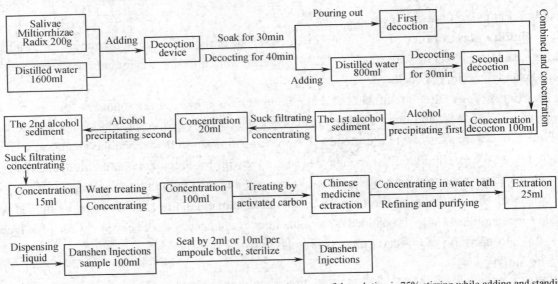

First alcohl precipitation: Adding 100% ethanol until the alcohol content of the solution is 75%, stirring while adding, and standin for more than 40h.

Alcohol precipitation: Adding 100% ethanol until the alcohol content of the solution is 85%, stirring while adding, and standing for more than 40h.

Treat with water: Adding 10 times of distil water, stirring, standing and refrigerating for 24h, filtering with double-layer filter paper, and adjusting pH to 6.8~7.0 with 20% NaOH.

Treat with activated carbon: Adding 0.2% activated carbon, boiling for 20min, filtering after slightly cooling.

Dispensing liquid: Add 0.3g sodium bisulfite, add water for injection to 100ml after dissolution.

Figure 6–1　The preparation procedure of injection (Danshen Injection)

【Characters】This product is a reddish-brown, clear liquid.

【Functions and Indications】Activating blood circulation and removing blood stasis. Used for angina pectoris and myocardial infarction caused by coronary artery insufficiency and myocardial anoxia.

【Usage and Dosage】Intramuscular injection, 2.0ml once, 1~2 times a day.

【Considerations】

(1) This product is a sterilized brown clear aqueous solution made of Radix Salviae Miltiorrhizae; each 1ml is equivalent to 2g of Salviae Miltiorrhizae Radix.

(2) Salviae Miltiorrhizae injection is TCMJ, and improper storage may affect the quality of the product. It must be light check before use. If finding that the solution is turbid, precipitated, discolored, leaked, or the bottle is slightly broken, it cannot be used.

(3) Salviae Miltiorrhizae injection should comply with the following relevant regulations during production and storage: ① It shall have no odor or rancidity odor; Unless otherwise specified, the color shall not be deeper than that of yellow No.6 standard colorimetric solution and shall keep transparency problem at 10°C. ② Iodine value is 79 ~ 128. The saponification value is 185~200. The acid value is not more than 0.56. Other solvents must be safe and harmless, and the dosage should not affect the curative effect.

(4) When preparing the injection, appropriate additives can be added according to the nature of the drug. If the additive is a bacteriostat, the dosage should be able to inhibit the growth of microorganisms in the injection. The commonly used bacteriostatic agent and dosage (g/ml) are 0.5% phenol, 0.3% cresol, 0.5% chlorobutanol, etc. Injections added with bacteriostats should still be sterilized by appropriate methods. If the injection volume exceeds 5ml, the added bacteriostatic agent must be especially carefully selected. No bacteriostat should be added to the injection for intravenous or spinal canal injection.

Unless otherwise specified, the containers shall conform to the provisions of the national standards on pharmaceutical glass containers. Container rubber plug shall comply with relevant regulations.

(5) When preparing the injection, the injected liquid medicine must be clear and the container should be clean and dry before use. When preparing the oil solution for injection, the refined oil should be first sterilized by dry heat at 150°C for 1~2 hours and then cooled to an appropriate temperature. Raw materials for direct sub-packaging into sterile powder for injection should be sterile. For powder obtained by freeze-drying, the liquid medicine prepared by using the powder should be sterile, and the difference in filling quantity should be controlled within ±4%.

(6) During the preparation process, the injection should be strictly prevent spoilage and contamination of microorganisms, pyrogens, etc. The dispensed solution should be sealed and sterilized within the same day. If it cannot be completed within the same day, the solution must be preserved under the condition of no deterioration and no easy propagation of microorganisms. Injections for intravenous and spinal canal injections should be more strictly controlled.

(7) The liquid is preserved under the condition of non-deterioration and non-breeding microorganism, and the injection for intravenous and spinal canal injection should be strictly controlled.

(8) When filling drugs that easily spoiled when exposed to air, the air in the container should be removed, filled with carbon dioxide or nitrogen and other gases, and then sealed the container.

(9) After the container is sealed or sealed tightly, the appropriate sterilization method can be selected according to the nature of the drug. The sterility of the finished product must be ensured.

(10) During or after sterilization, decompression method or other suitable methods shall be adopted for leak detection of the sealed injection.

(11) Injections shall be stored under light shielding according to specified conditions.

（V）Quality Inspection of Injection

1. Filling The volume of injections and liquid concentrates for injection should comply with the following requirements in the following test.

Procedure: Take 5 containers (the labeled quantity is not more than 2ml);take 3 containers (the labeled quantity should be more than 2ml and less than 50ml). Open the containers with caution to avoid any loss of the contents. Take up individually the contents of each container into a dry syringe, then discharge the contents of the syringe into a calibrated graduated cylinder (of such size that the volume to be measured should be at least 40% of its rated volume) and the measure takes place at room temperature. For injections of oily liquids or suspensions, warm-up and thoroughly shake the containers before removing the contents.Cool to room temperature before measuring the volume following the process as mentioned above.Each container is not less than the labeled quantity of the injection.

2. Weight variation　Unless otherwise specified, the weight variation of powders for injection should comply with requirements in the following test.

Procedure: take 5 sampled vials, remove any adherent label and the aluminum cap from the sealed container, wash the outside with ethanol and dry thoroughly, and weigh each container accurately and immediately. Open the container with caution to avoid foreign matter such as glass debris falling into the vial [Note: For powder formulations, caution need to betaken when removing the inner stopper (with consideration of air pressure change that may cause loss), and weigh the whole container immediately with inner stopper]. Remove the contents, wash the container thoroughly with water or ethanol, dry it in a suitable condition and weigh again.

Calculate the weight of the content in each container as well as the average value from 5 containers. The weight variation of the contents from each container does not deviate from the average weight by a percentage greater than that shown in the Table 6-1. If the weight variation of contents of one container does not comply with the above requirements, repeat the operation with another 10 containers, all of them should comply with the requirements.

Table 6-1　Limits of loading differences "*Chinese Pharmacopoeia*"

Average or labeled	Limit of loading difference
0.05g and below	±15%
Above 0.05g to 0.15g	±10%
Above 0.15 to 0.50g	±7%
0.50g or more	±5%

Generally, if the test for uniformity of content is specified for a sterilized powder for injection the lest for weight variation is not required.

3. Osmolality　Unless otherwise specified, the injections for intravenous infusions or vertebral injections should comply with the requirements of the determination of osmolality (General rule 0632) as specified in the individual monograph.

4. Visible particles　Unless otherwise specified, comply with the requirements of the test for visible particles in injections (General rule 0904).

5. Particulate matter　Unless otherwise specified, the examination of the solution-type injection for intravenous injection, intravenous drip, intrathecal injection, intraspinal injection, sterile powder for injection and concentrated solution for injection according to the insoluble particle inspection method (General rule 0903) shall comply with the regulations.

6. Chinese Medicine injection related substances　According to the provisions of the varieties, it should comply with the requirements of the Chinese Medicine injection related substances (General rule 2400).

7. Residual quantity of heavy metals and harmful elements　Unless otherwise specified, it should comply with the requirements of the test for lead, cadmium, arsenic, mercury, copper (General rule 2321) determination. According to the maximum daily use of the variety of calculation, the lead should no exceed 12μg, cadmium should no exceed 3μg, arsenic should no more than 6μg, mercury should not exceed 2μg, copper should not exceed 150μg.

8. Sterility　Comply with the requirements of the test for sterility (General rule 1101).

9. Bacterial endotoxin or pyrogens　Unless otherwise specified, the injections for intravenous infusions should comply with the requirements of the test for bacterial endotoxin(General rule 1143) or the test for pyrogens (General rule 1142) as a specified individual monograph.

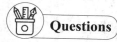 **Questions**

1. What are the main problems of TCM injections, how to deal with?

2. What are the types and varieties of additives commonly used in injections? What are the principles for selecting additives in injections?

3. What else are the preparation methods of the stock solution for TCM injection? What is the basis for the "water-alcohol method" to prepare TCM injections?

4. What are the differences in formulation preparation between traditional Chinese medicine injection and chemical injection?

PPT

实验七　软膏剂和乳膏剂的制备

 实验目的

1. **掌握**　不同类型软膏剂和乳膏剂的制备方法、关键操作和注意事项。
2. **熟悉**　药物加入基质中的方法以及不同类型基质对药物释放的影响。
3. **了解**　软膏剂和乳膏剂的质量检查方法。

实验提要

1. 软膏剂系指原料药物与油脂性或水溶性基质混合制成的均匀半固体外用制剂。乳膏剂系指原料药物溶解或分散于乳状液型基质中形成的均匀半固体制剂。软膏剂、乳膏剂主要对皮肤、黏膜或创面起保护、润滑和局部治疗作用，如消炎、杀菌防腐、收敛等。

2. 基质为软膏剂、乳膏剂的赋形剂，占软（乳）膏组成的大部分，基质对软（乳）膏剂的质量、理化特性及药物疗效的发挥均有极其重要的影响。

软膏剂的基质主要包括以下两类。

（1）油脂性基质　包括烃类、类脂类、动植物油脂类等，常用的有凡士林、羊毛脂、硬脂酸等。

（2）水溶性基质　由天然或合成的水溶性高分子物质组成，常用的有甘油、明胶、聚乙二醇等。

乳膏剂的基质为乳状液型基质，常用的乳化剂可分为水包油型和油包水型。水包油型乳化剂有钠皂、三乙醇胺皂类、聚山梨酯类等；油包水型乳化剂有钙皂、羊毛脂、单甘油酯等。

3. 不同类型软（乳）膏的制备可根据药物和基质的性质、制备量及设备条件不同而分别采用研和法、熔合法和乳化法制备。

（1）研和法　适用于基质较软，在常温下通过研磨即能与药物均匀混合，或不宜加热、不溶性及少量药物的制备。

（2）熔合法　若基质熔点不同，在常温下不能与药物均匀混合，多采用熔合法。

（3）乳化法　是制备乳膏剂的专用方法。将处方中油溶性组分一起加热至80℃左右，另将水溶性组分溶于水中，加热至80℃左右，两相混合，搅拌至乳化完全并冷凝。大量生产时，使用乳匀机或胶体磨可使产品更细腻均匀。

4. 不同类型的软（乳）膏基质对药物释放、吸收的影响不同，可用凝胶扩散法测定软（乳）膏中药物的释放性能。一般情况下，乳状液型基质的乳膏和水溶性基质的软膏释药较快，油脂性基质的软膏释药较慢。软（乳）膏剂除外观性状应符合质地均匀细腻、易涂布、色泽均匀一致、稠度适宜、无刺激性、无酸败等质量要求外，还需对药物的含量、软（乳）膏剂的物理性质、刺激性、稳定性及药物的释放、穿透及吸收进行评定。

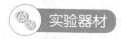　**实验器材**

1. **仪器**　恒温水浴锅、天平、蒸发皿、量筒、温度计、研钵、软膏刀等。
2. **试药**　黄芩苷细粉、凡士林、羊毛脂、冰片、硬脂酸、单硬脂酸甘油酯、蓖麻油、甘油、三乙醇胺、甲基纤维素、苯甲酸钠、紫草、当归、防风、地黄、白芷、乳香、没药、蜂蜡、蒸馏水。

　实验操作步骤

（一）软膏剂、乳膏剂的制备

1. 油脂性基质黄芩苷软膏

【**处方**】

黄芩苷细粉	0.8g
凡士林	17.4g
羊毛脂	1.8g

【**制法**】称取凡士林，加入羊毛脂，水浴（60℃）加热熔融后，加入黄芩苷细粉充分搅匀，放冷即得。

实验流程图如图 7-1 所示。

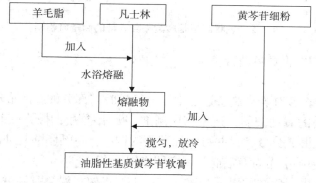

图 7-1　油脂性基质黄芩苷软膏的制备流程图

【**性状**】本品为均匀的淡黄色软膏。

【**注意事项**】油脂性基质黄芩苷软膏制备过程中，羊毛脂因过于黏稠而不宜单用，常与凡士林合用，以改善凡士林的吸水性和渗透性；药物加入熔化基质后，应不停搅拌至冷凝，否则药物分散不匀，但已凝固后应停止搅拌，否则空气进入膏体使软膏不能久贮。

2. 乳状液型基质黄芩苷乳膏

【**处方**】

黄芩苷细粉	0.8g
冰片	0.04g
硬脂酸	2.40g
单硬脂酸甘油酯	0.80g
蓖麻油	4.00g
甘油	2.00g
三乙醇胺	0.30ml
蒸馏水	10.00ml

【制法】

（1）将硬脂酸、单硬脂酸甘油酯、蓖麻油共置于干燥烧杯内，水浴加热至80℃，使全熔。

（2）将甘油、黄芩苷、蒸馏水置另一烧杯中，水浴加热至80℃，边搅拌边加入三乙醇胺，使黄芩苷全溶。

（3）将冰片加入（1）中溶解。

（4）立即将（1）逐渐加入（2）中，边加边搅拌均匀，至室温，即得。

实验流程图如图7-2所示。

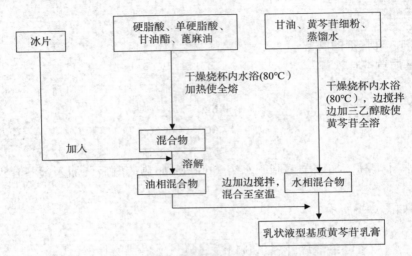

图7-2　乳状液型基质黄芩苷乳膏的制备流程图

【性状】 本品为均匀的橙黄色乳膏。

【注意事项】

（1）乳状液型基质黄芩苷乳膏制备过程中，三乙醇胺与部分硬脂酸形成硬脂酸胺皂，为O/W型乳化剂。硬脂酸胺皂的碱性较弱，适于药用制剂。硬脂酸用量中仅一部分与碱反应生成肥皂，未皂化的硬脂酸被乳化形成分散相，并可增加基质的稠度。单硬脂酸甘油酯能增加油相的吸水能力，在O/W型乳化剂基质中作为稳定剂并有增稠作用。

（2）在乳膏的制备中，应注意以下关键操作：①油水两相混合时温度应相同；②油、水、胶三者的混合顺序，初乳是否形成直接关系到最终成品的质量；③两相混合后，一般应沿一个方向不停搅拌，并注意搅拌速度，以免过快产生气泡，过慢乳化不完全或使药物析出；④冷凝后就应停止搅拌，以免带入气泡。

3. 水溶性基质黄芩苷软膏

【处方】

黄芩苷细粉	0.8g
甲基纤维素	3.4g
甘油	2.0g
苯甲酸钠	0.02g
蒸馏水	140ml

【制法】

（1）将黄芩苷细粉、苯甲酸钠置蒸发皿中，加入适量蒸馏水，水浴加热使溶解，放冷。

（2）另将甲基纤维素、甘油在研钵内研匀。

（3）将（1）加入到（2）中，边研边加，研匀即得。

实验流程图如图7-3所示。

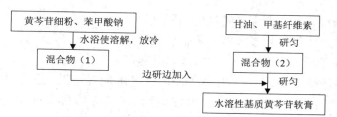

图 7-3　水溶性基质黄芩苷软膏的制备流程图

【性状】本品为淡黄色凝胶状软膏。

注释：①三种不同基质的黄芩苷软膏均为均匀、细腻、具有适当黏稠性的黄色半固体。②黄芩苷软膏有抗菌、消炎、抗过敏作用。三种不同基质软膏适应证有所不同，油膏主要适用于干燥创面；乳膏、水膏可用于有渗出液的皮肤病。

4. 紫草膏

【处方】

紫草	10g
当归	3g
防风	3g
地黄	3g
白芷	3g
乳香	3g
没药	3g
蓖麻油	100g
蜂蜡	适量
共制成150g	

【制法】

（1）原料处理　将乳香、没药粉碎成细粉，过七号筛。当归、防风、地黄、白芷酌予碎断；紫草用清水润湿。

（2）炸料制膏　取蓖麻油置于锅内，加热至约200℃，先将当归、防风、地黄、白芷4味药炸枯，至白芷表面呈焦黄色，除去药渣，降温至约160℃，再将紫草加入，用微火炸枯，至油呈紫红色，滤除药渣，加入蜂蜡适量（药油每10g，加蜂蜡约4g）熔化，倾入容器内，待温度降至60~70℃时，加入乳香、没药细粉，共制成150g，搅匀至冷凝，即得。

实验流程图如图 7-4 所示。

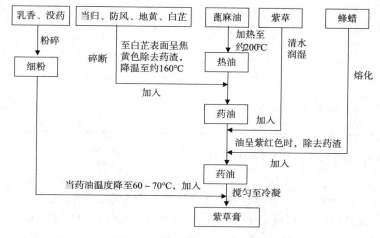

图 7-4　紫草膏的制备流程图

【性状】本品为紫红色的软膏，具特殊的油腻气。

【功能与主治】化腐生肌。用于疮疡、痈疽已溃等症。

【用法与用量】摊于纱布上贴患处，每隔1~2日换药一次。

【注意事项】紫草膏制备过程中，紫草应先用少量水润湿再投入药油中，否则会因温度过高而使紫草素破坏；操作中应注意防止着火，油温达到200℃后立即离火。

（二）软膏剂和乳膏剂中药物释放性能考察

1. 林格溶液的配制

【处方】

氯化钠	0.85g
氯化钾	0.03g
氯化钙	0.048g
蒸馏水	加至100ml

【制法】取氯化钠、氯化钾、氯化钙置100ml量筒中，加适量蒸馏水溶解，加蒸馏水定容至100ml，搅拌均匀即得。

2. 含指示剂的琼脂凝胶的制备

【处方】

琼脂	2g
林格氏溶液	120ml

【制法】称取琼脂2g，加入120ml林格化溶液内，水浴加热溶解，趁热用纱布滤过，冷至60℃，加入$FeCl_3$试液3ml，混匀，立即沿管壁小心倒入内径一致的三支相同试管（10ml）内，防止产生气泡，装量为距离口径10mm处，直立静置使凝固，备用。

3. 软膏剂和乳膏剂释放性能考察

实验步骤（一法）：将制得的3种不同基质的黄芩苷软（乳）膏，用软膏刀分别装满试管（与管口齐平），注意软膏应与琼脂表面密切接触，不留空隙。观察经一定时间药物向琼脂中渗透的距离（即变色的长度），将测得的数据填入表7-1内并绘制曲线，比较不同基质中药物释放的速度。

表7-1　不同基质黄芩苷软（乳）膏药物释放性能测定结果

时间 /h	扩散色区长度 /mm		
	油脂性基质	乳状液型基质（O/W型）	水溶性基质
1			
2			
4			
8			
16			
24			
K			

扩散距离与时间的关系可用以下公式表示：

$$Y^2 = K \times t$$

式中，Y为扩散距离，mm；t为扩散时间，h；K为扩散系数，mm^2/h。

以不同时间扩散色区的长度的平方（Y^2）对扩散时间（t）作图，可得一条直线，其斜率为K，K值大小反映软膏剂中药物释放能力的大小。

实验步骤（二法）：将以上配好的黄芩苷软（乳）膏 2g 均匀涂在载玻片上，放入培养皿中，加入 40ml 蒸馏水，经 2 分钟后，自培养皿中吸取 1ml 溶液加三氯化铁试液 1 滴，观察颜色变化，以溶液变色时记为药物开始释放的时间，比较药物在不同基质中的释放速度。

（三）软膏剂、乳膏剂的质量检查

1. 粒度 除另有规定外，混悬型软膏剂、含饮片细粉的软膏剂照下述方法检查，应符合规定。

检查法 取供试品适量，置于载玻片上涂成薄层，薄层面积相当于盖玻片面积，共涂 3 片，照粒度和粒度分布测定法（通则 0982 第一法）测定，均不得检出大于 180μm 的粒子。

2. 装量 照最低装量检查法（通则 0942）检查，应符合规定。

3. 无菌检查 用于烧伤［除程度较轻的烧伤（Ⅰ度或浅Ⅱ度）外］或严重创伤的软膏剂与乳膏剂，照无菌检查法（通则 1101）检查，应符合规定。

4. 微生物限度 除另有规定外，照非无菌产品微生物限度检查：微生物计数法（通则 1105）和控制菌检查法（通则 1106）及非无菌药品微生物限度标准（通则 1107）检查，应符合规定。

思考题

1. 本实验中采取了哪几种方法制备软膏剂？
2. 软膏剂制备中加入药物时，应注意哪些事项？
3. 乳膏剂制备时，水相和油相混合的先后顺序如何判断？
4. 分析药物在三种不同基质中的释放情况。

题库

Experiment 7 Preparation of Ointments and Creams

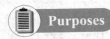

Purposes

1. To master the preparation methods, key operations and precautions of different types of ointments and creams.

2. To be familiar with the method of adding drugs to the bases and the effects of different types of bases on drug release.

3. To understand the quality inspection methods of ointments and creams.

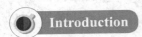

Introduction

1. Ointments are uniform semi-solid preparations made of drug substances and oleaginous or water-soluble bases and are intended for external application to the skin. Creams are uniform semi-solid preparations made of emulsion-type bases in which raw material drugs are dissolved or dispersed. Ointments and creams mainly play the roles of protection, lubrication and local treatment on skin, mucous membrane or wound such as anti-inflammation, sterilization, anticorrosion, convergence, etc.

2. The bases are the excipients of ointments and creams, which accounts for most of their composition. It has an extremely important effect on the quality, physical and chemical properties and curative effect of ointments (creams).

The bases of ointments mainly includes the following two categories:

(1) Oleaginous bases   Including hydrocarbons, lipids, animal and vegetable oils, etc., commonly used are vaseline, wool fat, stearic acid and so on.

(2) Water-soluble bases   It is composed of natural or synthetic water-soluble polymers, such as glycerin gelatin and polyethylene glycol, etc.

The bases of creams are emulsion, and the commonly used emulsifiers can be divided into water-in-oil type and oil-in-water type. Oil-in-water emulsifiers include sodium soap, triethanolamine soap and polysorbate, etc.; Oil-in-water emulsifiers are calcium soap, wool fat and monoglyceride, etc.

3. The different types of ointments and creams can be prepared by methods of leavigation, fusion and emulsification respectively according to the differences of drugs and bases properties, preparation quantity and equipment conditions.

(1) Leavigation   It is used for the bases which are soft and can be evenly mixed with drugs by leavigating at room temperature, or other bases which are not suitable for heating, insoluble and preparation with a small amount of drugs.

(2) Fusion   If the melting point of the bases is different, it cannot be uniformly mixed with the drug at room temperature, and at this time the fusion method is often used.

(3) Emulsification   It is a special method for the preparation of creams. In this method, the oil-

62

soluble components in the prescription are heated to about 80℃, and the water-soluble components are dissolved in water and heated to about 80℃, then the two phases are mixed and stirred until emulsified and condensed. In the large-scale production, the use of emulsion homogenizer or colloid mill can make the products more delicate and uniform.

4. Different types of bases have different effects on drug release and absorption of ointments and creams, and the drug release performance can be determined by gel diffusion method. Normally, the release of creams with emulsion-type bases and ointments with water-soluble bases is faster, while the release of ointments with oleaginous bases is slower. In addition to the appearance characteristics of ointments (creams), which should be consistent with the quality requirements of fine consistency, easy to coat, uniform color, moderate viscosity, no irritation and no rancidity, etc., concentrations, physical properties, irritation, stability, release, penetration and absorption of the drug should also be evaluated.

 Equipments and Materials

1. Equipments Thermostat water bath, balance, evaporating dish, measuring cylinder, thermometer, mortar, spatula, etc.

2. Materials Baicalin powder, vaseline, wool fat, borneol, stearic acid, glyceryl monostearate, castor oil, glycerine, triethanolamine, methylcellulose, sodium benzoate, Arnebiae Radix, Angelicae Sinensis Radix, Saposhnikoviae Radix, Rehmanniae Radix, Angelicae Dahuricae Radix, Frankincense, Myrrha, beeswax, distilled water.

 Experimental Procedures

（Ⅰ）Preparation of Ointments and Creams

1. Baicalin Ointments with oleaginous base

【Formula】

Baicalin powder	0.8g
Vaseline	17.4g
Wool fat	1.8g

【Preparation】Melt the vaseline and wool fat together in a water bath (60℃), add the fine powder of baicalin to the mixture and stir until baicalin is evenly dispered, and finally remove the mixture from the water bath and stir until congealed.

Experiment flow chart (Figure 7-1):

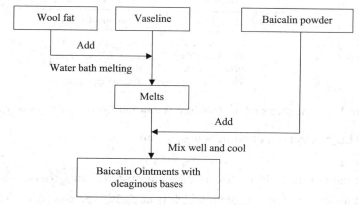

Figure 7-1 The preparation procedure of Baicalin Ointments with oleaginous base

【Characters】This product is an even ointments in faint yellow.

【Considerations】In the preparation of baicalin ointments with oleaginous bases, wool fat is too thick to be used alone and it is often used with vaseline to improve the water absorption and permeability of vaseline; After the addition of drug into the melting matrix, it should be continuously stirred until condensation, or the drug will not be evenly dispersed. However, stirring should be stopped after it has solidified, otherwise the air will enter the paste and the ointments can not be stored for long time.

2. Baicalin Creams of emulsion-type bases

【Formula】

Baicalin powder	0.8g
Borneol	0.04g
Stearic acid	2.40g
Glyceryl monostearate	0.80g
Castor oil	4.00g
Glyceryl	2.00g
Triethanolamine	0.30ml
Distilled water	10.00ml

【Preparation】

(1) Put stearic acid, glyceryl monostearate and castor oil in a dry beaker and heat to 80℃ in a water bath to dissolve completely.

(2) Put glycerin, baicalin powder, distilled water into another beaker, and heat to 80℃ in a water bath. Then add triethanolamine with stirring until the baicalin is completely dissolved.

(3) Add borneol to (1) to dissolve.

(4) Immediately add the phase (1) to the phase (2), stir while adding, and stir until the mixture cool to room temperature. The Baicalin Cream of emulsion-type bases is obtained.

Experiment flow chart (Figure 7–2):

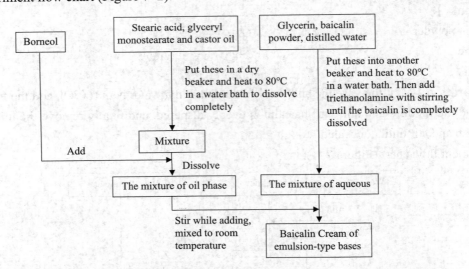

Figure 7–2　The preparation procedure of Baicalin Cream of emulsion-type bases

【Characters】This product is a uniform orange cream.

【Considerations】

(1) In the preparation of the Baicalin Cream of emulsion-type bases, triethanolamine forms a stearic acid amine soap with a portion of stearic acid, which is an O/W type emulsifier. The alkaline of stearic

acid amine soap is weak, which is suitable for pharmaceutical preparations. Only a portion of the stearic acid is reacted with alkali to form a soap, and others are emulsified to form a dispersed phase, thereby increasing the consistency of the bases. Glyceryl monostearate could increase the water absorption capacity of the oil phase and acts as a stabilizer in the O/W emulsifier bases with a thickening effect.

(2) In the preparation of creams, the following key operations should be noted: ①Oil phase and aqueous phase should be mixed at the same temperature; ②The order of mixing oil, aqueous and glue, and whether the primostrum could be formatted are directly related to the quality of the final product; ③After mixing the two phases, generally, stirring should be carried out in one direction, and pay attention to the stirring speed. Stir faster could generate bubbles, on the contrary, causing incomplete emulsification or drug precipitation; ④Stop stirring after condensation to avoid air bubbles.

3. Baicalin Ointments with water-soluble bases

【Formula】

Baicalin powder	0.8g
Methylcellulose	3.4g
Glycerin	2.0g
Sodium benzoate	0.02g
Distilled water	140ml

【Preparation】

(1) Put baicalin and sodium benzoate in the evaporating dish, add an appropriate amount of distilled water, heat in a water bath to dissolve and cool.

(2) Put methylcellulose, glycerin in the mortar grind evenly.

(3) Add (1) to (2), grind while adding, grind evenly.

Experiment flow chart (Figure 7−3):

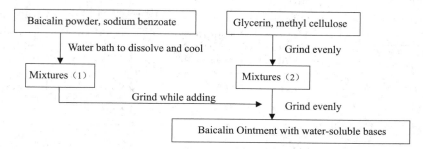

Figure 7−3　The preparation procedure of Baicalin Ointment with water-soluble bases

【Characters】This product is pale yellow gelatinous ointments.

Considerations: ①Baicalin ointments of three different bases are uniform, fine and yellow semi-solid with appropriate viscosity. ②Baicalin ointments have an antibacterial, anti-inflammatory, anti-allergic effect. Three different bases ointments indications are different, ointments are mainly used for drying wound; Cream, water cream can be used for skin diseases with exudate.

4. Zicao Ointments

【Formula】

Arnebiae Radix	10g
Angelicae Sinensis Radix	3g
Saposhnikoviae Radix	3g

Rehmanniae Radix	3g
Angelicae Dahuricae Radix	3g
Frankincense	3g
Myrrha	3g
Castor Oil	100g
Ceraflava	q.s.

Make a total of 150g

【Preparation】

(1) Raw material process   Crush frankincense and myrrha into fine powder and pass through No. 7 sieve. Angelicae Sinensis Radix, Saposhnikoviae Radix, Rehmanniae Radix, and Angelicae Dahuricae Radix are broken; Arnebiae Radix is moistened with water.

(2) Ointments are made of frying material   Take castor oil in a pot and heat it to about 200℃. Firstly, the four herbs of Angelicae Sinensis Radix, Saposhnikoviae Radix, Rehmanniae Radix, Angelicae Dahuricae Radix are fried dry until the surface of Angelicae dahurian is burnt yellow, remove the dregs, cool it to about 160℃, then add the Arnebiae Radix, fry it dry with low fire until the castor oil is purplish red, filter the dregs, add an appropriate amount of ceraflava (about 4g for medicine oil per 10g), melt it, and pour it into the container until the temperature drops to 60~70℃, add frankincense and myrrha powder to make a total amount of 150g, stir well while it condenses.

Experiment flow chart (Figure 7-4):

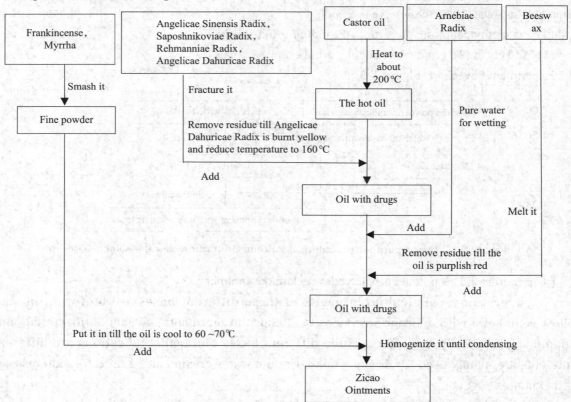

Figure 7-4   The preparation procedure of Zicao Ointments

【Characters】It is a purplish red ointment with special greasy smell.

【Functions and Indications】Remove necrosis and promote granulation for pyocutaneous, ulcer and etc.

【Usage and Dosage】Spread it on the gauze and stick it to the affected part with a change 1~2 days.

【Considerations】Arnebiae Radix should be wetted with a little water before being put in the oil in case of destroying Shikonin by excessive temperature. Fire protection should be noted. Oil should be taken away from heat sources till 200°C.

(Ⅱ) Investigate on Drug Release Performance of Ointments and Creams

1. Prepare Ringer's solution

【Formula】

NaCl	0.85g
KCl	0.03g
CaCl₂	0.048g
Distilled water	Add to 100ml

【Preparation】Put NaCl/ KCl/ CaCl$_2$ into a measuring cylinder (100ml) and add some distilled water to dissolve them. Then make the solution to 100ml and mix well.

2. Prepare agar gel containing the indicator

【Formula】

Agar	2g
Ringer's solution	120ml

【Preparation】Put agar 2g into Ringer's solution 120ml and heat in water-bath to dissolve. Filter with gauze while hot and mix with FeCl$_3$ 3ml well till cool to 60°C. Immediately pour carefully into 3 identical tubes (10ml) with the same inner diameter along the tube wall to make the level 10mm from the nozzle and stand it upright to solidify for future use. Be careful to prevent bubbles.

3. Investigate on release performance of ointments and creams

Experimental steps (method one): Fill the test tube with 3 kinds of baicalin ointments/creams with ointments knife to flush with a nozzle. It should be closely contacted to agar surface without gap. Observe the penetration distance (i.e. the length of discoloration) of drugs into agar after a certain period, fill data into the Table 7−1 and draw the curve, and compare the release rates.

Table 7−1 Determination of drug release properties of baicalin ointments/creams with different bases

Time/h	Diffusion color region length/mm		
	Oleaginous Bases	Emulsion-type Bases (O/W)	Water-soluble Bases
1			
2			
4			
8			
16			
24			
K			

The relationship between diffusion distance and time can be expressed by the following formula:

$$Y^2 = K * t$$

Where, Y is diffusion distance, mm; t is diffusion time, h; K is diffusion coefficient, mm^2/h.

Using the square of the length of different time diffusion color region (Y^2) to plot the diffusion time (t), a straight line can be obtained, the slope of which is K, and the value of K reflects the drug release ability in the ointments.

Experimental steps (method two): The above-mixed baicalin ointments/creams 2g was evenly coated on the slide, put it into the petri dish, add 40ml distilled water, after 2min, absorb the 1ml solution from the petri dish and add 1 drop of ferric trichloride test solution, and observe the color change. The discoloration of the solution was recorded as the starting time of drug release, and the release rates of drugs in different substrates were compared.

（Ⅲ）Quality Inspection of Ointments and Creams

1. Particle size　For suspended ointments and creams containing powders of prepared slices, unless otherwise specified, should comply with the following requirement.

Procedure: Spread a number of ointments onto three microscope slides separately to form a thin layer of which the area is equivalent to that of the cover-glass. Carry out the determination of particle size and particle size distribution (General rule 0982, method 1), no particle of greater than 180μm in dimension should be observed.

2. Filling　Comply with the test of minimum fill (General rule 0942).

3. Sterility　Ointments and creams for burns (Except for minor burns of 1st or minor 2nd degree) or grievous injuries should comply with the test of sterility (General rule 1101).

4. Microbial limit　Unless otherwise provided, ointments and creams should comply with microbiological examination of nonsterile products: microbial enumeration tests (General rule 1105), microbiological examination of nonsterile product: tests for specified microorganisms (General rule 1106) and microbiological acceptance criteria of nonsterile pharmaceutical products (General rule 1107).

 Questions

1. What methods have been used to prepare ointments in this experiment?
2. What matters should be paid attention to when adding drugs to the ointments?
3. How to judge the sequence of mixing water phase and oil phase in the preparation of creams?
4. Analyze drug releasing degree in three different bases.

实验八 栓剂的制备

实验目的

1. **掌握** 热熔法制备栓剂的方法和操作要点。
2. **熟悉** 栓剂基质的分类、栓剂置换价的计算及栓剂质量的检查方法。

实验提要

1. **定义** 栓剂系指原料药物与适宜基质制成供腔道给药的固体制剂。其形状与重量因使用腔道而异，常用栓剂有肛门栓和阴道栓。其栓模如图 8-1 所示。

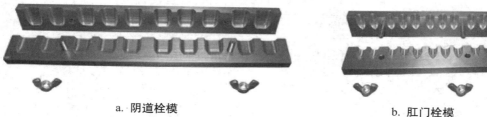

a. 阴道栓模
a. Vaginal suppository

b. 肛门栓模
b. Rectal suppository

图 8-1 栓模
Figure 8-1 Bolt mold

一般来说，固体药物应先用适宜方法制成极细粉，与油脂性基质混合。油溶性药物可直接混入已熔化的油脂性基质中，使之溶解，如果加入的药物量过大时能降低基质的熔点或使栓剂过软，可加适量石蜡或蜂蜡调节。水溶性药物，如中药浸膏，可直接与已溶化的水溶性基质混合，也可制成干浸膏粉与油脂性基质混合。

2. **制备方法** 栓剂的制法有搓捏法、冷压法、热熔法三种。其中热熔法最为常用，其制备工艺流程图如图 8-2 所示。

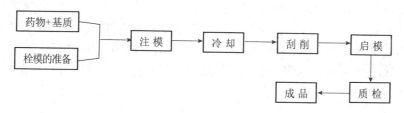

图 8-2 栓剂的制备工艺流程图

3. **基质** 栓剂常用的基质有油脂性基质、水溶性及亲水性基质等，应根据药物性质及治疗要求选用。为了使栓剂冷却后易从栓模中脱出，同时保证栓剂外观质量，栓剂应涂润滑剂。基质不同润滑剂不同。水溶性、亲水性基质的栓剂常用液状石蜡、植物油；油脂性基质的栓剂则用软肥皂、甘油各一份与 90% 乙醇 5 份制成的醇溶液。

实验器材

1. **仪器** 肛门栓模、阴道栓模、蒸发皿、七号筛、电炉、分析天平、融变时限检查仪。
2. **试药** 甘油、硬脂酸钠、三黄粉、冰片、半合成脂肪酸酯。

实验操作步骤

1. 甘油栓

【处方】

甘油	9.1g
硬脂酸钠	0.9g

【制法】取甘油置蒸发皿内，水浴加热，缓缓加入干燥的硬脂酸钠细粉，不断搅拌，并保温在 85~95℃，直至溶液澄清，滤过，注入涂过润滑剂（液状石蜡）的栓模中，冷却成型，脱模，即得。

实验流程图如图 8-3 所示。

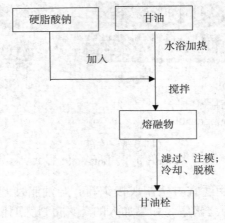

图 8-3 甘油栓的制备工艺流程图

【注意事项】

（1）钠肥皂（硬脂酸钠）为硬化剂，吸收甘油而成固体凝胶。由于肥皂的刺激和甘油较高的渗透压，故能增加肠的蠕动而显泻效。

（2）制备时必须避免温度过高，搅拌不宜太快，否则引入气泡，使成品混浊不澄明。

（3）优良的栓剂应具有一定的硬度，无刺激性，引入腔道后熔融或软化，外形应整齐美观，其内外颜色应一致。本品为无色或几乎无色的透明或半透明栓，适用于各种便秘，尤其适用于小儿及年老体弱者，每次一支。

2. 三黄栓

【处方】

三黄粉	2g
冰片	0.2g
半合成脂肪酸酯	8g

【制法】将半合成脂肪酸酯粉碎成粗末，水浴加热至熔（40℃以下），加入三黄粉、冰片，搅

匀注入涂有润滑剂（肥皂醑）的栓模中，凝固后整理脱模，取出栓剂，即得。

实验流程图如图 8-4 所示。

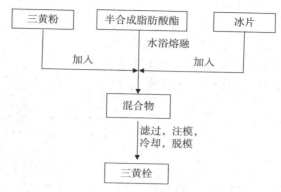

图 8-4　三黄栓的制备流程图

【注意事项】

（1）半合成脂肪酸酯类熔点低，熔距短，抗热性好，贮存较稳定，熔点 35~37℃，水浴锅 40℃ 即可。

（2）冰片具易挥发性，水浴温度不可过高。

（3）本品为褐黄色栓剂，清热解毒，消炎，用于治疗肛窦炎、肛乳头炎、直肠炎、痔瘘术后预防感染、便秘等，一次一枚，一日 1~2 次。

3. 融变时限检查　仪器装置由透明的套筒与金属架组成（图 8-5a）。

透明套筒为玻璃或适宜的塑料材料制成，高为 60mm，内径为 52mm，及适当的壁厚。

金属架由两片不锈钢的金属圆板及 3 个金属挂钩焊接而成（图 8-5b）。每个圆板直径为 50mm，具 39 个孔径为 4mm 的圆孔；两板相距 30mm，通过 3 个等距的挂钩焊接在一起。

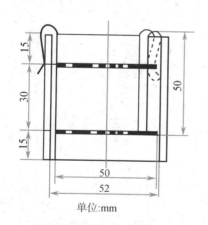
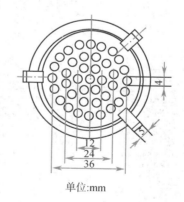

a. 透明套筒与金属架　　　　　　　　b. 金属架结构
a. Transparent sleeve and mental frame　　**b. Mental frame structure**

图 8-5　融变时限检查装置

取供试品栓剂 3 粒，在室温放置 1 小时后，照《中国药典》2020 年版四部融变时限检查法检查，油脂性基质的栓剂 3 粒应在 30 分钟内全部融化、软化或触压时无硬心；水溶性基质的栓剂 3 粒应在 60 分钟内全部溶解。如有 1 粒不合格，应另取 3 粒复试，均应符合规定。

题库

思考题

1. 热熔法制备栓剂应注意什么问题？如何评价栓剂的质量？

2. 甘油栓的制备原理及操作时的注意事项是什么？

3. 制备栓剂时测定药物对基质的置换价有何意义？

Experiment 8 　Preparation of Suppositories

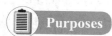
Purposes

　1. To master the method and main points of hot melt preparation of suppositories.

　2. To be familiar with the classification of suppository matrix, the calculation of suppository replacement value and the method of checking suppository quality.

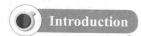
Introduction

　1. Meaning　Suppositories are solid preparations made by the drug substance and a suitable matrix for intraluminal administration. Its properties and weight vary depending on the cavity used. Anal and vaginal suppositories are commonly used suppositories. The bolt mold is shown in the Figure 8–1.

　Generally, solid drugs should be made into extremely fine powders by suitable methods and mixed with an oil-soluble matrix. The oil-soluble drug can be directly mixed into the melted oily matrix to dissolve it. If the amount of the drug added is too large, it can lower the melting point of the matrix or make the suppository too soft, and it can be adjusted by adding an appropriate amount of paraffin or beeswax. Water-soluble drugs, such as traditional Chinese medicine extracts, can be directly mixed with the dissolved water-soluble matrix, or they can be made into dry soaking powder and mixed with a greasy matrix.

　2. Preparation method　There are three methods for preparing suppositories: kneading method, cold pressing method and hot-melt method. Among them, the hot melt method is the most commonly used, and its preparation process is (Figure 8–2):

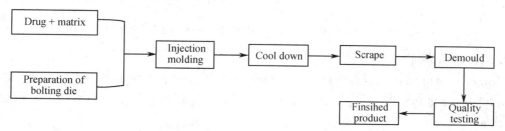

Figure 8–2　The preparation procedure of suppositories

　3. Matrix　The commonly used matrices of suppositories are greasy matrix, water-soluble and hydrophilic matrix, etc., which should be selected according to the nature of the drug and treatment requirements. In order to make the suppository easy to come out of the suppository after cooling, and at the same time to ensure the appearance quality of the suppository, the suppository should be coated with a lubricant. Different lubricants are used for different substrates. Water-soluble, hydrophilic base

73

suppositories are usually liquid paraffin and vegetable oil; oily base suppositories are alcoholic solutions made of soft soap, one part of glycerin and five parts of 90% ethanol.

Equipments and Materials

1. Equipments Anal plug mold, vaginal plug mold, evaporating dish, No.7 sieve, electric furnace, analytical balance, fusion time limit checker

2. Materials Glycerin, sodium stearate, Sanhuang powder, borneol, semi-synthetic fatty acid ester.

Experimental Procedures

1. Glycerin Suppository

【Formula】

Glycerin	9.1g
Sodium stearate	0.9g

【Preparation】Take glycerin in an evaporation dish, heat it in a water bath, slowly add dry sodium stearate powder, keep stirring, and keep it at 85-95°C until the solution is clear, filter, and inject lubricant (liquid paraffin). In the bolt mold, cooling molding and demoulding are obtained.

Experiment flow chart (Figure 8-3):

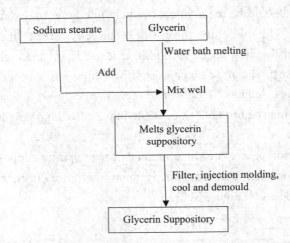

Figure 8-3 The preparation procedure of Glycerin Suppository

【Considerations】

(1) Sodium soap (sodium stearate) is a hardener that absorbs glycerin to form a solid gel. Due to the irritation of soap and the osmotic pressure of glycerol, it can increase the peristalsis of the intestine and show a laxative effect.

(2) During the preparation, the temperature must be avoided to be too high, and the stirring should not be too fast, otherwise air bubbles will be introduced to make the finished product cloudy and unclear.

(3) An excellent suppository should have a certain hardness and no irritation. It should be melted or softened after being introduced into the cavity, and its appearance should be neat and beautiful, and its internal and external colors should be consistent.This product is a colorless or almost colorless transparent

or translucent suppository, suitable for all kinds of constipation, especially for children and elderly frail people, one at a time.

2. **Sanhuang Shuan**

【 Formula 】

Sanhuang powder	2g
Borneol	0.2g
Semi-synthetic fatty acid ester	8g

【 Preparation 】 Crush the semi-synthetic fatty acid ester into coarse powder, heat it in the water bath to melt (below 40°C), add Sanhuang powder and borneol, stir and inject into the suppository mold coated with lubricant (soap tincture). After solidification, open the mold, remove the suppository. That's it.

Experiment flow chart (Figure 8-4):

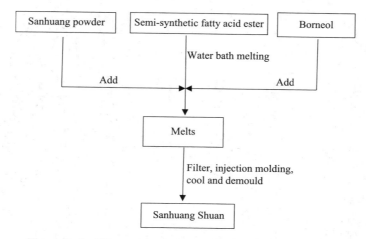

Figure 8-4 The preparation procedure of Sanhuang Shuan

【 Considerations 】

(1) Semi-synthetic fatty acid lipids have low melting point, short melting distance, good heat resistance, stable storage, melting point $35 \sim 37°C$, water bath pot 40°C.

(2) Borneol is volatile, and the temperature of the water bath must not be too high.

(3) This product is a brown-yellow suppository, clearing away heat and detoxifying, anti-inflammatory, for the treatment of anal sinusitis, anal papillitis, proctitis, postoperative hemorrhoid fistula infection prevention, constipation, etc., one at a time, 1~2 times a day.

3. **Melt time limit test**   The device consists of a transparent sleeve and a metal frame (Figure 8-5a).

The transparent sleeve is made of glass or suitable plastic material, with a height of 60mm, an inner diameter of 52mm, and an appropriate wall thickness.

The metal frame is welded by two stainless steel metal plates and three metal hooks (Figure 8-5b). Each circular plate is 50mm in diameter and has 39 circular holes with a hole diameter of 4mm; the two plates are 30mm apart and are welded together by 3 equidistant hooks.

Take 3 test suppositories, and leave them at room temperature for 1 hour, and check according to the *Chinese Pharmacopoeia's* fusion time limit inspection method. The 3 suppositories of the greasy matrix should all be melted, softened or touched within 30 minutes. There is no hard heart; suppositories of water-soluble matrix should be completely dissolved within 60 minutes. If there is one grains of suppository that does not conform to the requirements, another three capsules should be taken for retesting, all of which should meet the requirements.

 Questions

1. What should be paid attention to when preparing suppositories by hot melt method? How to evaluate the quality of suppositories?

2. What is the preparation principle and precautions of glycerin suppository?

3. What is the significance of determining the replacement value of the drug to the matrix when preparing suppositories?

PPT

实验九 丸剂的制备

实验目的

1. **掌握** 不同类型丸剂的制备方法、关键操作和注意事项。
2. **熟悉** 水丸、蜜丸、滴丸对药物和辅料的处理原则及各类丸剂的质量要求。
3. **了解** 滴丸的制备原理及影响滴丸质量的因素。

实验提要

1. 丸剂系指原料药物与适宜的辅料制成的球形或类球形固体制剂，中药丸剂包括蜜丸、水丸、糊丸、蜡丸、浓缩丸和滴丸等，化学药丸剂包括滴丸、糖丸等。

2. 蜜丸系指饮片细粉以炼蜜为黏合剂制成的丸剂。其中每丸重量在 0.5g（含 0.5g）以上的称大蜜丸，每丸重量在 0.5g 以下的称小蜜丸。水丸系指饮片细粉以水（或根据制法用黄酒、醋、稀药汁、糖液、含 5% 以下炼蜜的水溶液等）为黏合剂制成的丸剂。滴丸系指原料药物与适宜的基质加热熔融混匀，滴入不相混溶、互不作用的冷凝介质中制成的球形或类球形制剂。

3. 不同类型丸剂的制备可根据药物和基质的性质、制备量及设备条件不同，而采用泛制法、塑制法或滴制法。

（1）泛制法 在泛丸机中交替撒布药粉与润湿剂，使药粉润湿、翻滚、黏结成粒，逐渐增大成丸的一种制丸方法，可用于水丸、水蜜丸、浓缩丸、糊丸的制备。其制备工艺流程图如图 9-1 所示。

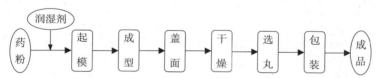

图 9-1 泛制法制备工艺流程图

（2）塑制法 饮片细粉与适宜黏合剂（常用炼蜜）制成软硬适宜的丸块，再经过制丸条、制丸粒等工序制备丸剂的方法，可用于蜜丸、水蜜丸、浓缩丸、糊丸、蜡丸的制备。其制备工艺流程图如图 9-2 所示。

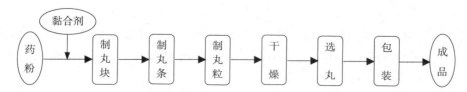

图 9-2 塑制法制备工艺流程图

（3）滴制法 系指中药提取物或有效成分与适宜的基质加热熔融，混合均匀，滴入与之不相混溶的冷凝剂中，冷凝成丸的方法，用于滴丸剂的制备。其制备工艺流程图如图 9-3 所示。

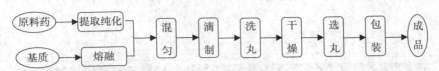

图 9-3　滴制法制备工艺流程图

4. 水丸制备时，根据药料性质、气味等可将药粉分层泛入丸内，以掩盖不良气味，防止芳香成分的挥发损失。也可将速效部分泛于外层，缓释部分泛于内层，达到长效的目的。一般选用黏性适中的药物细粉起模，并应注意掌握好起模用粉量。如用水为润湿剂，必须用 8 小时以内的凉开水或蒸馏水。盖面时要特别注意分布均匀。

5. 除另有规定外，供制丸剂用的药粉应为细粉或最细粉。炼蜜按炼蜜程度分为嫩蜜、中蜜和老蜜，制备时可根据品种、气候等具体情况选用。蜜丸应细腻滋润，软硬适中。

6. 滴丸基质包括水溶性基质和非水溶性基质，常用的有聚乙二醇类（如聚乙二醇 6000、聚乙二醇 4000 等）、泊洛沙姆、硬脂酸聚烃氧（40）酯、明胶、硬脂酸、单硬脂酸甘油酯、氢化植物油等。滴丸冷凝介质必须安全无害，且与原料药物不发生作用。常用的冷凝介质有液状石蜡、植物油、甲基硅油和水等。

实验器材

1. **仪器**　水浴锅、不锈钢托盘、搓丸板、搓条板、瓷盘、烧杯、温度计、电炉、滴丸机、天平、崩解仪、七号筛等。

2. **试药**　防风等饮片、蜂蜜、聚乙二醇 6000（PEG 6000）、硬脂酸、二甲基硅油、包装纸等。

实验操作步骤

（一）丸剂的制备

1. 防风通圣丸

【处方】

防风	5g	荆芥穗	2.5g
薄荷	5g	麻黄	5g
大黄	5g	芒硝	5g
栀子	2.5g	滑石	30g
桔梗	10g	石膏	10g
川芎	5g	当归	5g
白芍	5g	黄芩	10g
连翘	5g	甘草	20g
白术（炒）	2.5g		

【制法】以上十七味，除芒硝、滑石外，其余防风等15味粉碎成细粉，过筛，混匀。芒硝加水溶解，滤过；将滑石粉碎成极细粉，备用。取上述已混匀粉末，用芒硝滤液泛丸，干燥，用滑石粉包衣，打光，干燥，即得。

实验流程图如图 9-4 所示。

【性状】本品为包衣或不包衣的水丸，丸芯呈浅棕色至黑褐色；味甘、咸、微苦。

【功能与主治】解表通里，清热解毒。用于外寒内热，表里俱实，恶寒壮热，头痛咽干，小便短赤，大便秘结，瘰疬初起，风疹湿疮。

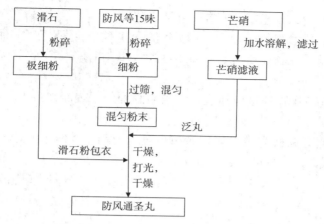

图 9-4　防风通圣丸的制备流程图

【用法与用量】口服。水丸一次 6g，一日 2 次；浓缩丸一次 8 丸，一日 2 次。

【注意事项】

（1）可以粉末直接起模、湿颗粒起模，也可以用混浆起模，所得模核应过二号筛。

（2）成型即是将筛选均匀的丸模反复加水润湿，撒粉，滚圆至成品规格。每次加水，加粉量要适宜，分布要均匀。

（3）及时挑出过大或过小丸粒，并将其用水调成药液，以混浆喷入。若有发生黏丸或黏锅，可加入少许干粉并搅拌。

2. 大山楂丸

【处方】

山楂	50g
六神曲（麸炒）	7.5g
炒麦芽	7.5g

【制法】以上三味，分别粉碎成细粉，过七号筛，混匀；另取蔗糖 30g，加水 13ml 与炼蜜 30g，混合，炼至相对密度约为 1.38（70℃）时，滤过，与上述粉末混匀，制丸块，搓丸条，制丸粒，每丸重 9g，即得。

实验流程图如图 9-5 所示。

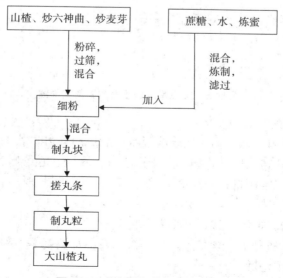

图 9-5　大山楂丸的制备流程图

【性状】本品为棕红色或褐色的大蜜丸；味酸、甜。

【功能与主治】开胃消食。用于食积内停所致的食欲不振，消化不良，脘胀腹闷。

【用法与用量】口服。一次 1~2 丸，一日 1~3 次，小儿酌减。

【注意事项】

（1）搓丸条与分丸粒操作速度应适宜。丸条粗细均匀，表面光滑无裂缝，内部充实无裂隙，以便分粒和搓圆。

（2）制丸时应在上下搓板沟槽中均匀涂布少量润滑剂（香油：蜂蜡 =10 : 2~3），以防粘连，并使丸粒表面光滑。成丸后立即分装，不须干燥。

（3）蜜丸极易染菌，应采取恰当措施和方法，防止微生物污染。根据药物的性质采用适宜的灭菌方法。

3. 穿心莲内酯滴丸

【处方】

穿心莲内酯	1.0g
聚乙二醇 6000	17.5g
硬脂酸	0.75g

【制法】

（1）取聚乙二醇 6000 置蒸发皿中，于水浴上加热至全部熔融，加入穿心莲内酯及硬脂酸，搅拌至熔化。

（2）将熔融的药液转移至滴丸机贮液器中，通入 80~85℃ 循环水保温，打开贮液器下端开关，调节滴出口与冷却剂间的距离，控制滴速为每分钟 30~50 滴，待滴丸完全冷却后，取出滴丸。

（3）摊于滤纸上，擦去表面附着的液状石蜡（或二甲基硅油），装于瓶中，即得。每粒重 40mg。

实验流程图如图 9-6 所示。

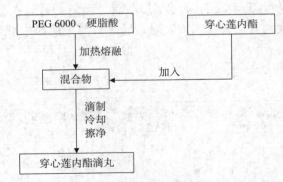

图 9-6　穿心莲内酯滴丸的制备流程图

【性状】本品为类白色滴丸，味苦。

注释：本品为二萜类内酯化合物，均难溶于水，制成滴丸可显著提高生物利用度。

【功能与主治】芳香开窍，理气止痛。用于冠心病、胸闷、心绞痛、心肌梗死等。

【用法与用量】口服。常用量，一次 2~4 粒，一日三次。发病时可含服或吞服。

【注意事项】

（1）滴丸应大小均匀，色泽一致，不得发霉变质。

（2）滴丸的成型与基质种类、含药量、冷却液以及冷却温度等多种因素有关。

（二）丸剂的溶散时限考察

取供试品 6 丸，选择筛网孔径适当的吊篮（丸剂直径在 2.5mm 以下的用孔径约 0.42mm 的筛网；在 2.5~3.5mm 之间的用孔径约 1.0mm 的筛网；在 3.5mm 以上的用孔径约 2.0mm 的筛网），启动崩解仪进行检查。小蜜丸、水蜜丸和水丸应在 1 小时内全部溶散；浓缩水丸和糊丸应在 2 小时内全部溶散。滴丸不加挡板检查，应在 30 分钟内全部溶散，包衣滴丸应在 1 小时内全部溶散。操作过程中当供试品粘附挡板妨碍检查时，应另取供试品 6 丸，不加挡板进行检查。上述检查中供试品应在规定时间内全部通过筛网。如有细小颗粒状物未通过筛网，但已软化且无硬心，可按符合规定论。结果可填入表 9-1。

除另有规定外，大蜜丸及研碎、嚼碎后或用开水、黄酒等分散后服用的丸剂不检查溶散时限。

表 9-1 不同丸剂溶散时限检查结果

品种	溶散时限 /min	检查结果 /min	是否符合规定
防风通圣丸	60		
大山楂丸	/		
穿心莲内酯滴丸	30		

（三）丸剂的质量检查

1. **外观**　丸剂外观应圆整均匀、色泽一致。大蜜丸和小蜜丸应细腻滋润，软硬适中。滴丸应大小均匀，色泽一致，表面的冷凝液应除去。

2. **水分**　照水分测定法（《中国药典》2020 年版（四部）测定，除另有规定外，大蜜丸、小蜜丸、浓缩蜜丸中所含水分不得过 15.0%；水蜜丸、浓缩水蜜丸不得过 12.0%；水丸、糊丸和浓缩水丸不得过 9.0%；蜡丸不检查水分。

3. **重量差异**　按（《中国药典》2020 年版四部）制剂通则丸剂项下测定。

4. **装量**　照最低装量检查法（通则 0942）检查，应符合规定。

5. **微生物限度**　除另有规定外，照非无菌产品微生物限度检查：微生物计数法（通则 1105）和控制菌检查法（通则 1106）及非无菌药品微生物限度标准（通则 1107）检查，应符合规定。

思考题

1. 本实验中采取了哪几种方法制备丸剂？
2. 如何炼制蜂蜜？为什么要炼蜜？
3. 请简述水丸起模的方法与操作要点。
4. 影响滴丸成型的因素有哪些？

题库

Experiment 9 　Preparation of Pills

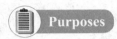

Purposes

1. To master the preparation methods, key operations and precautions of different types of pills.

2. To be familiar with the treatment principles of watered pills, honeyed pills and dripping pills for medicine materials and auxiliary materials and the quality requirements of various pills.

3. To understand the preparation principles of dripping pills and the factors affecting the quality of dripping pills.

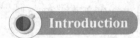

Introduction

1. Pills are spherical or quasi-spherical solid preparations made of raw materials and appropriate auxiliary materials. Chinese medicine pills include honeyed pills, watered pills, paste pills, wax pills, concentrated pills, dripping pills, etc., while chemical pills include dripping pills, sugared pills, etc.

2. Honeyed pills refer to the pill made of the fine powder of the decoction pieces and the honey refining as the adhesive. Each pill with a weight of more than 0.5g (including 0.5g) is called big honeyed pills, and each pill with a weight of less than 0.5g is called small honeyed pills. Watered pills are made of water (or rice wine, vinegar, thin medicine juice, sugar solution, water solution containing less than 5% honey refining, etc.) as the adhesive for the fine powder of decoction pieces. Dripping pills are spherical or quasi-spherical preparations made by heating and melting the raw material medicine and the suitable matrix, and dropping it into the immiscible and non-interacting condensing medium.

3. Based on the properties of drugs and matrix, the amount of preparation and the conditions of equipment, the preparation process of different types of pills is categorized as rubbing method, moulding method and dripping method, respectively.

(1) Rubbing method is a method for preparing watered pills, honeyed pills, concentrated pills and paste pills, by alternately spreading powder and adhesive in the pan pill machine to make the powder wet, tumble, stick and gradually increase into pills. The preparation process is shown in the Figure 9–1.

(2) Moulding method can be used for the preparation of honeyed pills, water honeyed pills,

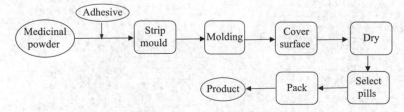

Figure 9–1　Preparation process flow of rubbing method

82

concentrated pills, paste pills and wax pills. The method of making soft and hard pellets with fine powder of decoction pieces and suitable adhesive (commonly used to make honey), and then preparing pellets through the processes of pill making, pill making, etc. The preparation process is shown in the Figure 9–2.

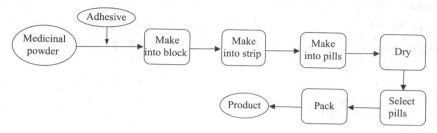

Figure 9–2   Preparation process flow of moulding method

(3) Dripping method refers to the method for the extract or effective component of traditional Chinese medicine, by heating and melting with the appropriate matrix and mixing evenly, to be dropped into the immiscible condensing agent and then condensing into pills. Dripping method is used for the preparation of dripping pills, and the preparation process is shown in the Figure 9–3.

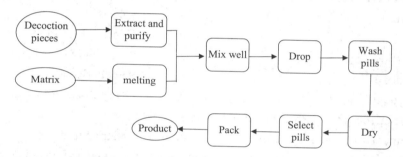

Figure 9–3   Preparation process flow of dripping method

4. During the preparation of watered pills, according to the nature and smell of the drug, the powder can be layered into the pills to cover up the bad smell and prevent the loss of volatile components. The quick-acting part can also be extended to the outer layer and sustained-release part to the inner layer to achieve the long-term purpose. Generally, the fine powder with moderate viscosity is selected for mould lifting, and the amount of powder used for mold lifting should be well controlled. If water is used as wetting agent, it must be boiled or distilled water within 8 hours. Special attention should be paid to even distribution when covering.

5. Unless otherwise specified, the powder used for pill making should be the fine powder or the finest powder. Honey refining can be divided into tender honey, medium honey and old honey according to the degree of honey refining. It can be selected according to the variety, climate and other specific conditions during preparation. Honeyed pills should be delicate and moist, moderate in hardness and softness.

6. The drop pills matrix includes water-soluble matrix and non-water-soluble matrix. The commonly used drop pills are polyethylene glycol (such as polyethylene glycol 6000, polyethylene glycol 4000, etc.), poloxamer, stearic polyoxy (40) ester, gelatin, stearic acid, glycerin monostearate, hydrogenated vegetable oil and other cold coagulation media, which must be safe and harmless, and have no effect on the raw materials. The common condensing media are liquid paraffin, vegetable oil, methyl silicone oil and water, etc.

Equipments and Materials

1. Equipments   Water bath pot, stainless steel tray, pill rolling plate, strip rolling plate, porcelain plate, beaker, thermometer, electric furnace, pill dropping machine, balance, disintegrator, No.7 sieve, etc.

2. Materials   Saposhnikoviae Radix and other decoction pieces, honey, PEG 6000, stearic acid, dimethylsilicone oil, packaging paper, etc.

Experimental Procedures

（Ⅰ）Preparation of Pills

1. Fangfeng Tongsheng Pill

【Formula】

Saposhnikoviae Radix	5g	Schizonepetae Spica	2.5g
Menthae Haplocalycis Herba	5g	Ephedrae Herba	5g
Rhei Radix Et Rhizoma	5g	Natrii Sulfas	5g
Gardeniae Fructus	2.5g	Talcum	30g
Platycodonis Radix	10g	Gypsum Fibrosum	10g
Chuanxiong Rhizoma	5g	Angelicae Sinensis Radix	5g
Paeoniae Radix Alba	5g	Scutellariae Radix	10g
Forsythiae Fructus	5g	Glycyrrhizae Radix Et Rhizoma	20g
Atractylodis Macrocephalae Rhizoma (Fried)	2.5g		

【Preparation】The above seventeen flavors, in addition to Natrii Sulfas and Talcum, the other 15 flavors such as Saposhnikoviae Radix are crushed into fine powder, sifted and mixed evenly. Natrii Sulfas dissolved in water and filtered. The talcum powder is crushed into a very fine powder and set aside. Natrii Sulfas filtrateis used to pan pill, followed by drying, coating with talcum powder, polishing and drying again.

Experiment flow chart (Figure 9–4):

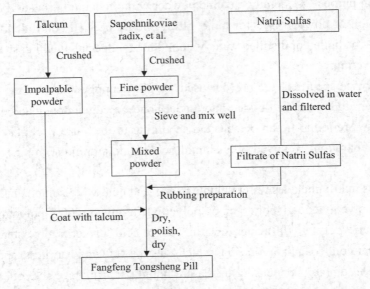

Figure 9–4   The preparation flow chart of Fangfeng Tongsheng Pill

【Characters】This product is coated or uncoated watered pill. The core color of the pill is light brown to dark brown. It tastes sweet, salty and slightly bitter.

【Functions and Indications】Remove the exterior, clear away the heat and detoxify the interior. It is used for external cold and internal heat, exterior and interior solid, cold and strong heat, headache and dry throat, short and red urination, defecation secret knot, first onset of scrofula, rubella and wet sore.

【Usage and Dosage】Oral administration. 6g watered pills at a time, twice a day; 8 concentrated pills at a time, twice a day.

【Considerations】

(1) The mold can be directly lifted by powder, wet particles or mixed slurry. The obtained mold core shall pass No.2 sieve.

(2) Molding process is to add water repeatedly on the shot mold for wetting, dusting, rolling and screening. Each time water is added, the amount of powder added shall be appropriate and the distribution shall be uniform.

(3) Pick out the oversized or undersized pills in time, and mix them with water to form liquid medicine, and spray them into the mixture. If there is any sticky pill or pot, add a little dry powder and stir.

2. Big Hawthorn Pill

【Formula】

Crataegi Fructus	50g
Medicated Leaven (Stir-frying with bran)	7.5g
Fried Hordei Fructus Germinatus	7.5g

【Preparation】The above three flavors are crushed into fine powder separately, passed through sieve of No.7, and mixed evenly; in addition, take 30g of sucrose, add 13ml of water and 30g of refining honey, mix them, and when the relative density is about 1.38 (70℃), filter them, mix them with the above powder, make pellets, rub strips, and make pellets, each pill with the weight of 9g.

Experiment flow chart (Figure 9–5):

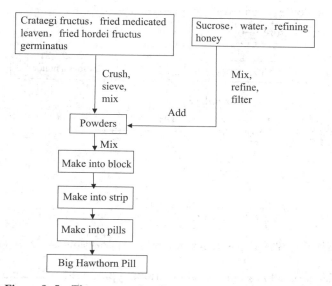

Figure 9–5   The preparation flow chart of Big Hawthorn Pill

【Characters】This product is brownish red or brown honeyed pill; it tastes sour and sweet.

85

【Functions and Indications】Appetizer and promote digestion. It is used for anorexia, dyspepsia and abdominal distention caused by food accumulation.

【Usage and Dosage】Oral. One or two pills at a time, one to three times a day, the dose for children shall be decreased accordingly.

【Considerations】

(1) The operation speed of rubbing strip and separating shot should be suitable. The bead is uniform in thickness, smooth on the surface and free of cracks. The inner part is full and free of cracks, so that it can be divided and rounded.

(2) A small amount of lubricant (balm: beeswax=10 : 2 ~ 3) shall be evenly coated in the grooves of upper and lower washboards during shot making to prevent adhesion and make the surface of shot smooth. After pelletizing, it should be repacked immediately without drying.

(3) Honeyed pills are easy to infect bacteria, so appropriate measures and methods should be taken to prevent microbial pollution. According to the nature of the drug, appropriate sterilization methods are used.

3. Andrographolide Dripping Pill

【Formula】

Andrographolide	1.0g
PEG 6000	17.5g
Stearic acid	0.75g

【Preparation】

(1) Put polyethylene glycol 6000 into an evaporating dish, heat it in the water bath until it is completely melted, add andrographolide and stearic acid, and stir until it is melted.

(2) Transfer the molten liquid medicine to the liquid accumulator of the dropping machine, put 80 ~ 85°C circulating water into it for heat preservation, turn on the lower switch of the liquid accumulator, adjust the distance between the dropping outlet and the coolant, control the dropping speed to 30 ~ 50 drops per minute, take out the dripping pill after the dripping pill is completely cooled.

(3) Spread it on the filter paper, wipe off the liquid paraffin (or dimethylsilicone oil) attached to the surface, and put it into the bottle. Each grain weighs 40mg.

Experiment flow chart (Figure 9–6):

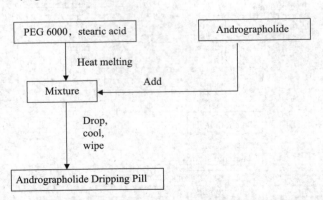

Figure 9–6　The preparation flow chart of Andrographolide Dripping Pill

【Characters】This product is a kind of white dripping pill, with bitter taste.

Note: The product is a diterpenoid lactone compound, which is difficult to dissolve in water. The preparation of dripping pill can significantly improve the bioavailability.

【Functions and Indications】It can open the orifices with fragrance, regulate qi and relieve pain. For coronary heart disease, chest distress, angina, myocardial infarction, etc.

【Usage and Dosage】Oral. Commonly used quantity: 2~4 capsules at a time, three times a day. Take or swallow when the disease occurs.

【Considerations】

(1) The pills should be uniform in size and color, and should not be moldy.

(2) The formation of dripping pills is related to many factors such as matrix type, drug content, coolant and cooling temperature.

(Ⅱ) Inspect the Dispersion Time of Pills

Take 6 pills from the test sample, select a basket with appropriate mesh diameter (the basket with a mesh diameter of about 0.42mm for pills with a diameter of less than 2.5mm; the sieve with a mesh diameter of about 1.0mm for pills with a diameter of 2.5~3.5mm; the sieve with a mesh diameter of about 2.0mm for pills with a diameter of more than 3.5mm), and start the disintegrator for inspection. Small honeyed pills, watered pills and watered-honeyed pills should be dispersed in 1 hour; concentrated watered pills and pasted pill should be dispersed in two hours. Dripping pills shall be dispersed completely within 30 minutes without baffle, and coated dripping pills shall be dispersed completely within 1 hour. In the process of operation, when the test object adheres to the baffle to hinder the inspection, another 6 pills of test object shall be taken for inspection without baffle. In the above inspection, all test objects shall pass through the screen within the specified time. If there are small particles that fail to pass the screen, but have softened and no hard core, it can be regarded as conforming to the regulations.

Unless otherwise specified, the dispersion limit of honeyed pills and pills taken after grinding, chewing or dispersing with boiled water, rice wine, etc. shall not be checked. The results are drawn as shown in the Table 9−1.

Table 9−1 Inspection results of dissolution limit of different pills

Varieties	Dispersion limit /min	Examination result /min	Compliance with regulations(Y or N)
Fangfeng Tongsheng Pill	60		
Big Hawthorn Pill	/		
Andrographolide Dripping Pill	30		

(Ⅲ) Quality Inspection of Pills

1. The appearance of pills shall be round and uniform with consistent color. Big honeyed pills and small honeyed pills should be delicate and moist, moderate in hardness and softness. The dripping pills shall be uniform in size and color, and the condensate on the surface shall be removed.

2. The water content shall be determined according to the water content determination method (*Chinese Pharmacopoeia*, 2020 Edition (Vol. Ⅳ)). Unless otherwise specified, the water content of big honeyed pills, small honeyed pill and concentrated honeyed pills shall not exceed 15.0%; the water content of water honeyed pill and concentrated honeyed pills shall not exceed 12.0%; the water content of watered pills, paste pill and concentrated watered pills shall not exceed 9.0%; the water content of wax pills shall not be checked.

3. The weight difference shall be determined according to the general principles of preparations (*Chinese Pharmacopoeia*, 2020 Edition (Vol. Ⅳ)).

4. The loading shall be inspected according to the minimum loading inspection method (General rule 0942), which shall meet the requirements.

5. Unless otherwise specified, microbial limit of non-sterile products shall be inspected according to microbial count method (General rule 1105), control bacteria inspection method (General rule 1106) and microbial limit standard of non-sterile drugs (General rule 1107), which shall meet the requirements.

 Questions

1. Which methods have been used to prepare pills in this experiment?
2. What are the methods or procedures of making honey? What are the purposes of making honey?
3. Please briefly describe the method and operation points of water shot mold lifting.
4. What are the factors influencing the formation of dripping pills?

实验十　颗粒剂的制备

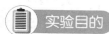 **实验目的**

1. **掌握**　颗粒剂的制备方法。
2. **熟悉**　颗粒剂的质量要求和质量检查方法。

实验提要

1. 颗粒剂系指药物与适宜的辅料混合制成具有一定粒度的干燥颗粒状剂型。按溶解性能和溶解状态分类，中药颗粒最常见的是可溶颗粒、混悬颗粒和泡腾颗粒三类。

2. 颗粒剂的制备主要包括原辅料的处理、制颗粒、干燥、整粒、分装等工序。

3. 处方原料药物的处理一般包括饮片浸提、浸提液纯化、浓缩或干燥等工艺过程。制备水溶颗粒时饮片多采用煎煮法浸提，也可根据饮片中活性成分的性质采用渗漉、浸渍或回流等浸提方法。含芳香挥发性活性成分的饮片一般以水蒸气蒸馏法提取挥发性成分备用，药渣煎煮提取。

浸提液的纯化可采用乙醇沉淀、高速离心（或与醇沉法联用）、大孔树脂吸附等方法。精制液可浓缩成适宜相对密度的稠浸膏，也可进一步干燥成干浸膏；或将精制液直接喷雾干燥制得浸膏粉，再行湿法或干法制粒。

4. 颗粒剂中常用的赋形剂有糖粉、糊精、乳糖等，以浸膏为原料制粒时，辅料的用量可根据浸膏的相对密度、黏性强弱等适当调整，但辅料总用量不宜超过清膏的 5 倍。以浸膏粉为原料制粒时，辅料的用量不宜超过浸膏粉量的 2 倍，湿法制粒时常选用适宜浓度的乙醇作为润湿剂。

5. 制粒是颗粒剂制备的关键工序，常用制粒方法有挤出制粒、湿法混合制粒、干法制粒等。湿颗粒制成后，应及时干燥。干燥温度应逐渐上升，一般控制在 60~80℃。

6. 处方中的挥发油常用适量的高浓度乙醇溶解后，喷洒于干颗粒中，密闭使均匀吸收。亦可将挥发油制成 β- 环糊精包合物，与干颗粒混合均匀。

实验器材

1. **仪器**　烧杯、烧瓶、颗粒筛、烘箱、天平、挥发油提取器。
2. **试药**　大青叶、板蓝根、连翘、拳参、荆芥穗、薄荷、防风、柴胡、紫苏叶、葛根、桔梗、苦杏仁、白芷、苦地丁、芦根、乙醇、蔗糖粉、糊精。

实验操作步骤

（一）感冒退热颗粒
【处方】

大青叶 100g　　　板蓝根 100g　　　连翘 50g　　　拳参 50g

【制法】

（1）煎煮　以上四味，加水煎煮两次，每次 1.5 小时，合并煎液，滤过。

（2）醇沉　将滤液浓缩至相对密度约为 1.08（90~95℃）的清膏，待冷至室温，加等量的乙醇使沉淀，静置。

（3）水沉　取上清液浓缩至相对密度为 1.20（60℃）的清膏，加等量的水，搅拌，静置 8 小时。

（4）制粒　取上清液浓缩成相对密度为 1.38~1.40（60℃）的稠膏，加蔗糖粉、糊精及乙醇适量，制成颗粒，干燥，整粒，分装（每袋装 18g），即得。

感冒退热颗粒制备的实验流程如图 10-1 所示。

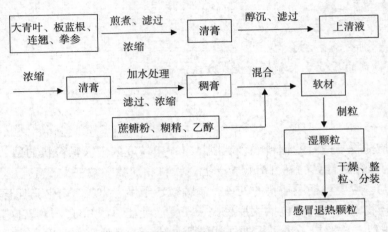

图 10-1　感冒退热颗粒的制备流程图

【性状】本品为棕黄色的颗粒，味甜、微苦。

【功能与主治】清热解毒，疏风解表。用于上呼吸道感染、急性扁桃体炎、咽喉炎属外感风热、热毒壅盛证，症见发热、咽喉肿痛。

【用法与用量】开水冲服。一次 1~2 袋，一日 3 次。

【规格】每袋装 18g。

【注意事项】

（1）制粒时选用 60%~70% 的乙醇作润湿剂制软材，不易粘连，便于操作。挤出制粒时软材的软硬程度对颗粒质量影响很大，应以"手握成团，轻压即散"为宜。

（2）清膏与赋形剂的用量比应视清膏的含水量而定，一般为 1:（2~4），总用量一般不超过清膏量的 5 倍。

（二）感冒清热颗粒

【处方】

荆芥穗 200g	薄荷 60g	防风 100g	柴胡 100g	紫苏叶 60g	葛根 100g
桔梗 60g	苦杏仁 80g	白芷 60g	苦地丁 200g	芦根 160g	

【制法】

（1）水蒸气蒸馏　以上十一味，取荆芥穗、薄荷、紫苏叶提取挥发油，蒸馏后的水溶液另器收集。

（2）煎煮　药渣与其余防风等八味加水煎煮两次，合并煎液，滤过，滤液与上述水溶液合并。

（3）软材制粒　合并液浓缩成相对密度为 1.32~1.35（50℃）的清膏。取清膏，加蔗糖粉、糊精及乙醇适量，制成颗粒，干燥，整粒，加入上述挥发油，混匀，分装（每袋装 12g），即得。

感冒清热颗粒制备的实验流程如图 10-2 所示。

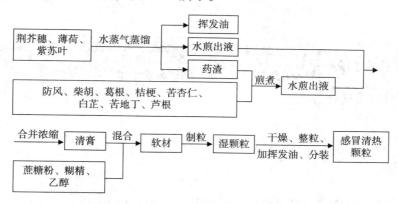

图 10-2　感冒清热颗粒的制备流程图

【**性状**】本品为棕黄色的颗粒，味甜、微苦。

【**功能与主治**】疏风散寒，解表清热。用于风寒感冒，头痛发热，恶寒身痛，鼻流清涕，咳嗽咽干。

【**用法与用量**】开水冲服。一次 1 袋，一日 2 次。

【**规格**】每袋装 12g。

【**注意事项**】荆芥穗、薄荷、紫苏叶含挥发油类有效成分，为避免挥发油在颗粒制备过程中受热挥发损失，采用水蒸气蒸馏法提取挥发油，待干颗粒整粒后，用少量高浓度乙醇溶解并喷洒于干颗粒中，密闭使均匀吸收。

（三）颗粒剂的质量检查

1. **粒度**　按照《中国药典》（2020 年版）测定，不能通过一号筛与能通过五号筛的总和不得过 15%。

2. **水分**　按照《中国药典》（2020 年版）总则中水分测定法测定，不得过 8.0%。

3. **溶化性**　取供试品 1 袋，加热水 200ml，搅拌 5 分钟，立即观察，应全部溶化，允许有轻微混浊。

4. **装量差异**　取供试品 10 袋，分别称定每袋内容物的重量，每袋装量与标示装量相比较，超出装量差异限度（±5%）的不得多于 2 袋，并不得有 1 袋超出限度 1 倍。

5. **微生物限度**　照《中国药典》（2020 年版）进行检查，应符合规定。

思考题

1. 常用的制粒方法有哪些？
2. 颗粒剂中常用的辅料有哪些？怎样合理选用辅料？
3. 采用挤出制粒法时，影响颗粒质量的主要因素有哪些？

题库

Experiment 10 Preparation of Granules

 Purposes

1. To master the preparation methods of granules.
2. To be familiar with the quality requirements and quality inspection methods of granules.

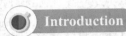 **Introduction**

1. Granule is a kind of dosage form with dry particle character, made by the mixture of medicine ingredient and appropriate excipients. According to its solubility and dissolution state, it could be classified as water-soluble granules, suspended granules and effervescent granules.

2. The main preparation approach of granule includes the pre-treatment of raw materials, granulation, drying, sort out granule, packaging, and so on.

3. The pre-treatment of raw materials generally includes a series of processes, such as the soaking extraction of decoction pieces, purification of extract solution, concentration or drying. To prepare the water-soluble granules, the decoction pieces are commonly extracted by decocting method, percolation, impregnation, or reflux method, based on the properties of contained active ingredients. Additionally, the decoction pieces containing volatile components are usually extracted by steam distillation primarily to obtain volatile components, and then boiling the decoction residue.

Secondly, the purification of the extract solution can be implemented by ethanol precipitation, high speed centrifugation or combined it with alcohol precipitation, macroporous resin adsorption and so on. After purification, the extraction solution could be concentrated as thick extractum with the suitable relative density, or be further dried into dry extract. Furthermore, the extraction solution could be directly dried into extract powder by spray drying, and then make granules by wet or dry granulation methods.

4. The commonly used excipients in granules are sugar powder, dextrin, lactose, etc. When the extractum is used as the raw material for granulation, the amount of excipients can be adjusted according to the relative density and viscosity of extractum. Nevertheless, the total amount of excipients should not exceed 5-fold of that of thin extract in that case. When extract powder is used as the raw material for granulation, the amount of excipients should not exceed 2-fold of that of extractives. Additionally, a certain amount of ethanol with suitable concentration is often used as wetting agent in wet granulation method.

5. Granulation is the key process of granule preparation. The common granulation methods include extrusion granulation, wet mixed granulation, dry granulation, etc. Among this approach, the wet granules should be dried in time with the gradually raising temperature ranging from 60 to 80℃.

6. Commonly, the volatile oil is usually dissolved in proper amount of high concentration ethanol,

then sprayed into the dry particles, and sealed aim to uniform absorption. Moreover, the volatile oil can also be encapsulated into β-cyclodextrin inclusion and mixed evenly with dry granules.

Equipments and Materials

1. Equipments　Beaker, flask, granule sieve, oven, electronic balance, volatile oil extractor, etc.

2. Materials　Isatidis Folium, Isatidis Radix, Forsythiae Fructus, Bistortae Rhizoma, Schizonepetae Spica, Menthae Haplocalycis, Saposhnikoviae Radix, Bupleuri Radix, Perillae Folium, Puerariae Lobatae Radix, Platycodonis Radix, Armeniacae Semen Amarum, Angelicae Dahuricae Radix, Corydalis Bungeanae Herba, Phragmitis Rhizoma, sucrose powder, dextrin, ethanol, etc.

Experimental Procedures

(I) Ganmao Tuire Granule

【Formula】

Isatidis Folium	100g
Isatidis Radix	100g
Forsythiae Fructus	50g
Bistortae Rhizoma	50g

【Preparation】

(1) Add the defined amount of water into the above four herbs, and decoct twice with each 1.5h.

(2) After filtration, the decoction solution for twice is merged and concentrated to a "thin extractum" with a relative density of about 1.08 (at 90~95℃). When the "thin extractum" was cool to room temperature, an equal quantity of ethanol was add to precipitate the impurities.

(3) The mixture was placed for standing for a while and filtered to collect the supernatant liquor, which was subsequently concentrated to a "thin extractum" with a relative density of about 1.20 (at 60℃). The obtained "thin extractum" was mixed with an equal quantity of water with stirring. After standing for 8h, the mixture was separated with different layers.

(4) The supernatant liquor is collected by filtration and concentrated to a "thick extractum" with a relative density of about 1.38~1.40 (at 60℃). After adding the defined amount of sucrose powder, dextrin and ethanol, granules were produced by extrusion granulation approach, with drying, sieving and packaging into single package of 18g in succession.

The experimental procedure for the preparation of Ganmao Tuire Granule is shown in the Figure 10-1 as following.

【Characters】This product is brownish-yellow granule with sweet / slightly bitter taste.

【Functions and Indications】To clear heat, remove toxin, dispel wind and relieve exterior syndrome. It is suitable for the treatment of upper respiratory tract infection, acute tonsillitis, and laryngopharyngitis, which are resulted from exogenous wind-hot, or accumulated heat-toxin, with the specific symptoms such as fever and swollen sore throat.

【Administration and Dosage】Taking the granules orally with hot water dispersion. 1~2 packages per time, and three times a day.

【Specification】18g per package.

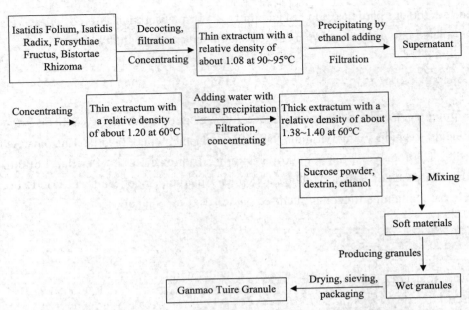

Figure 10-1　The preparation procedure of Ganmao Tuire Granule

【Considerations】

(1) During the granule preparation, 60% ~ 70% ethanol is used as wetting agent to make soft material, which is not easy to result in adhesion, but easy to operate. The degree of hardness and softness of soft material has a great influence on the granule quality in the process of extrusion granulation. The recommended state of soft material is to form block mass with hand holding and to disperse easily when gently pressing it.

(2) The weight ratio of thin extractum and excipients is generally 1:(2~4), according to the water content of thin extractum. The total amount of soft material cannot exceed 5-fold of the amount of thin extractum.

（Ⅱ）Ganmao Qingre Granule

【Formula】

Schizonepetae Spica	200g
Menthae Haplocalycis	60g
Saposhnikoviae Radix	100g
Bupleuri Radix	100g
Perillae Folium	60g
Puerariae Lobatae Radix	100g
Platycodonis Radix	60g
Armeniacae Semen Amarum	80g
Angelicae Dahuricae Radix	60g
Corydalis Bungeanae Herba	200g
Phragmitis Rhizoma	160g

【Preparation】

(1) Briefly, the volatile oil in Schizonepetae Spica, Menthae Haplocalycis, and Perillae Folium are extracted by steam distillation method. The aqueous solution of herbs after distillation was collected.

(2) And then, the herb residues of Schizonepetae Spica, Menthae Haplocalycis, and Perillae Folium, combined with the other eight herbs, were decocted twice with the defined amount of water. The extraction solution in twice decocting was merged, filtered and mixed with the above aqueous solution.

(3) The merged extraction solution was concentrated into a thin extractum with a relative density of about 1.32~1.35 (at 50℃). After adding the defined amount of sucrose powder, dextrin and ethanol, granules were produced by extrusion granulation approach, with drying, and sieving. After adding the volatile oil, granules are packaged into single package of 12g.

The experimental procedure for the preparation of Ganmao Qingre Granule is shown in the Figure 10-2 as following.

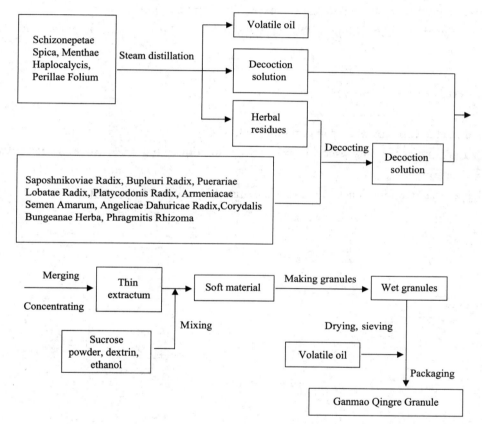

Figure 10-2   The preparation procedure of Ganmao Qingre Granule

【Characters】This product is brownish-yellow granule with sweet or slightly bitter taste.

【Functions and Indications】To dispel wind, remove cold, relieve exterior syndrome and clear heat. It is used for common cold due to wind-cold, with the symptoms such as headache and fever, cold aversion and bodily pain, turbid nasal discharge, cough and dry throat.

【Usage and Dosage】Taking the granules orally with hot water dispersion. 1 package per time, and twice a day.

【Specification】12g per package.

【Considerations】The volatile oil in Schizonepetae Spica, Menthae Haplocalycis, and Perillae Folium exhibits bioactive. Therefore, the volatile oil should be primarily extracted by steam distillation, in order to avoid the loss by heating during the granule preparation. And then, the volatile oil is dissolved in a small amount of high concentration ethanol and sprayed into the dry granules. With granules sealed, volatile oil could be evenly absorbed in granules.

(Ⅲ) Quality inspection of granules

1. Granularity   According to the current edition of *Chinese Pharmacopoeia*，the sum of not passing No.1 sieve and passing No.5 sieve should not exceed 15%.

2. Water content   According to the current edition of *Chinese Pharmacopoeia* in the general provision, the water content should not exceed 8%.

3. Dissolution   One bag of granules is added into 200ml of hot water with stirring for 5 minutes. Observe immediately, the granules should be completely dissolved, with slight turbidity allowed.

4. Loading variation   10 bags of granules are sampled. Each bag of granules is weighed. Compare the weight of each package with cthe labelled weight, no more than 2 bags are allowed to exceed the loading variation limit (±5%), and no bag can exceed the limit by 1 times.

5. Microbial limit   According to the current edition of *Chinese Pharmacopoeia*，it should meet the requirements.

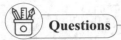

Questions

1. What are the commonly used granulating methods?

2. What are the commonly used excipients in granule preparation? How to select the variety of excipients reasonably?

3. What are the main influence factors for the granule quality in extrusion granulation?

实验十一 片剂的制备

PPT

实验目的

1. **掌握** 片剂的制备工艺及操作要点。
2. **熟悉** 片剂的质量要求与质量检查方法。
3. **了解** 压片机的基本构造及操作流程。

实验提要

1. 中药片剂系指原料药物或与适宜的辅料制成的圆形或异形的片状固体剂型。中药片剂按原料来源可分为提纯片、浸膏片、半浸膏片和全粉末片，其中半浸膏片所占比例最大。片剂制备工艺流程：物料准备 → 饮片处理（粉碎、提取、精制等）→ 制颗粒（湿法或干法）→ 干燥 → 整粒 → 压片 →（包衣）→ 质检 → 包装。

2. 中药原料应根据药物所含有效成分的性质进行浸提、分离、精制等处理，挥发性或遇热易分解的药物活性成分，在药料处理过程中应避免高温。用量极少的贵重药、毒性药，某些含少量芳香挥发性成分的饮片宜粉碎成细粉，过五至六号筛。

3. 片剂的辅料为片剂中除药物以外的物质的总称，包括稀释剂、吸收剂、润湿剂、黏合剂、崩解剂及润滑剂等。常用的稀释剂有淀粉、糖粉、糊精、乳糖等；常用的吸收剂有硫酸钙、碳酸钙等；常用的润湿剂为水和乙醇等；常用的黏合剂有淀粉浆、糖浆等。干淀粉、羧甲基淀粉钠等为常用的崩解剂；滑石粉、硬脂酸镁为常用的润滑剂。

4. 制颗粒是制备片剂的重要步骤。首先必须根据药物的性质选择润湿剂或黏合剂。制软材时要控制润湿剂或黏合剂的用量，使软材达到"握之成团、轻压即散"的程度。制粒时，应根据片重选择制粒筛。

5. 已制好的湿颗粒应根据药物和辅料的性质于适宜温度（60~80℃）干燥。对湿、热稳定的药物，干燥温度可适当提高。干燥后的颗粒需再进行过筛整粒，整粒时筛网孔径应与制粒用筛网孔径相同或略小。整粒后加入润滑剂、崩解剂等辅料，混匀，压片。

实验器材

1. **仪器** 单冲压片机、颗粒机、烘箱、乳钵、搪瓷盘、制粒筛、分析天平、硬度计、脆碎度测定仪、崩解时限测定仪。
2. **试药** 板蓝根、野菊花、土牛膝、贯众、氯苯那敏、滑石粉。

实验操作步骤

（一）感冒片的制备

【处方】

板蓝根	250g（粉料30g，膏料220g）
野菊花	125g（粉料50g，膏料75g）
土牛膝	125g（膏料）
贯众	125g（膏料）
氯苯那敏	125mg（粉料）
3%滑石粉	适量

【制法】

（1）粉料　研细，取过六号筛的板蓝根30g、野菊花50g，另放备用。

（2）膏料　取膏料药物饮片，置煎锅内，加6倍量水煮沸30分钟，滤过，药渣再加4倍量水煮沸30分钟，滤过，合并滤液，浓缩至约200ml。

（3）醇处理　根据浓缩液体积，加入适量乙醇，使含醇量达70%，冷藏静置24小时以上。

（4）浓缩收膏　吸去上清液，下层液抽滤，合并药液，减压回收至无醇味，移至适宜容器中，于100℃水浴上继续浓缩至约70g。

（5）混合粉料　将氯苯那敏研细过六号筛，与板蓝根、野菊花粉料混合均匀。

（6）制颗粒　将粉料置搪瓷盘内，加入热浸膏迅速拌匀，制成软材，制粒，颗粒摊于搪瓷盘内，置烘箱中60~70℃烘干，整粒。

（7）压片　按干颗粒重量加入3%的滑石粉，混匀，压片，即得。

实验流程图如图11-1所示。

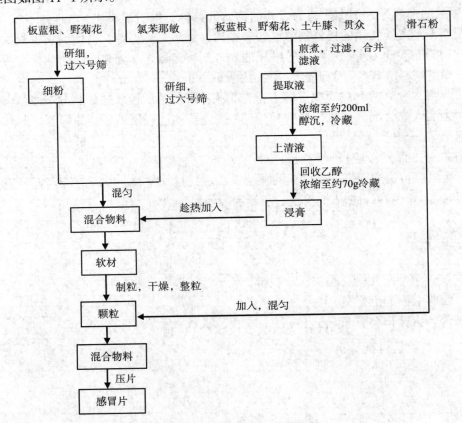

图11-1　感冒片的制备流程图

【**性状**】本品为棕色的半浸膏片，气香、味苦。

【**功能与主治**】清热解毒。用于感冒初起，恶寒发热、头疼鼻塞、咽喉肿痛等。

【**用法与用量**】口服，一次 4~6 片，一日 3 次。

【**注意事项**】中药半浸膏片可按中药饮片出膏率和出粉率，调整膏料与粉料的用量比例。

（二）片剂的质量检查

1. **外观检查**　应完整光洁，色泽均匀；应有适宜的硬度。

2. **重量差异**　除另有规定外，片剂的重量差异应符合规定（表 11-1）。

表 11-1　片剂重量差异限度

平均片重或标示片重	重量差异限度
0.30g 以下	± 7.5%
0.30g 及 0.30g 以上	± 5 %

检查法　取供试品 20 片，精密称定总重量，求得平均片重后，再分别精密称定每片的重量，每片的重量与平均片重相比较（凡无含量测定的片剂或有标示片重的片剂，每片重量应与标示片重比较），超出重量差异限度的不得多于 2 片，并不得有 1 片超过重量差异限度的 1 倍。

3. **崩解时限**　照崩解时限检查法（通则 0921）检查，应符合规定。一般半浸膏片的崩解时限为 60 分钟。

4. **硬度**　采用硬度计测定，应符合要求。

5. **脆碎度**　照片剂脆碎度检查法（通则 0923）检查，应无断裂、龟裂或粉碎片，片剂的减失重量一般不得超过 1%。

思考题

1. 制备片剂时为何要先制颗粒？
2. 如何决定中药半浸膏片中膏料和粉料的用量？
3. 影响片剂的硬度、崩解度和重量差异的因素有哪些？
4. 如何防止浸膏片吸潮？

题库

Experiment 11　Preparation of Tablets

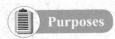 **Purposes**

1. To master the general preparation process and the key operating points of tablets.
2. To be familiar with the quality requirements and quality inspection methods of tablets.
3. To understand the basic structure and operation process of single punch tablet press.

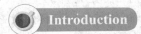 **Introduction**

1. Tablets are solid preparations of various shapes, round or heteromorphic, and obtained by compressing uniform volumes of particles consisting of drug substance with suitable excipients. Traditional Chinese medicinal tablets also include extract tablets, semi-extract tablets and powdered crude tablets, in which the semi-extract tablets are used most widely. The preparation process of tablets is as follows: Material preparation→Chinese medicine processing (crushing, extraction, purification, etc.)→make granulations (wet method or dry method)→drying→screen granulations→compressing tablets→(coating)→quality control→packaging.

2. Crushing, extraction, purification and other process should be carried out according to the active ingredients contained in the Chinese medicine raw materials. The volatile or heat-sensitive drugs should avoid high temperature in the medicine handling process. Dosage is very valuable drugs, toxic drugs, and some containing small amount of aromatic volatile components should be crushed into fine powders, and pass through No. 5 or No. 6 sieve.

3. The excipients are the materials included in the tablets prescription except drugs, such as diluents, absorbing agent, wetting agent, binder, disintegrating agent and lubricant, etc. The commonly used excipients of each kind are as follows: starch, sugar powder, dextrin and lactose for diluents, calcium sulfate and calcium carbonate for absorbing agents, water and ethanol for wetting agents, starch slurry and syrup for binders, dry starch and sodium carboxymethyl starch for disintegrating agents, talcum powder and magnesium stearate for lubricants.

4. Granulating in an important step in the process of tablets preparation. The choice of blinder and wetting agent should be based on the nature of drugs. The moisture content in the wet mass has a great influence on the quality of the resulting tablets, and is mostly judged by experience. The mass should be "forming a wet mass when holding and breaking up when pressing softly". The sieve for making granules should be chosen according to the weight of tablets.

5. The obtained wet granules should be dried at appropriate temperature (60~80℃) according to the nature of the drug and excipients. The dry temperature can be appropriately increased when drug is stable to wet or heat. The granules should be screened by passing through a suitable sieve, and the mesh size should be the same as the sieve used in the granulating process or slightly smaller. The lubricant,

disintegrating agents and other excipients were added after screening granules. Then mix them well and compress the mixture materials into tablets.

Equipments and Materials

1. Equipments　Single-punch press, granulator, oven, mortar, enamelled dish, granulating screen, electronic balance, tablet hardness tester, friabilator, disintegration time tester.

2. Materials　Isatidis Radix, Wild chrysanthemum, Achyranthes aspera, Cyrtomium fortunei, chlorphenamine, talcum powder.

Experimental Procedures

（Ⅰ）Preparation of Ganmao Tablets

【Formula】

Isatidis Radix	250g (powder 30g, extract 220g)
Wild chrysanthemum	125g (powder 50g, extract 75g)
Achyranthes aspera	125g (extract)
Cyrtomium fortunei	125g (extract)
Chlorphenamine	125mg (powder)
3% Talcum powder	q.s.

【Preparation】

(1) The fine powder of Isatidis Radix and Wild chrysanthemum is obtained by crushing raw materials over No. 6 sieve, before mixing well.

(2) Decoct the above four ingredients for 0.5h twice, the first time with the equivalent of 6 times the amount of water, and the second time with 4 times the amount of water. Then filter, combine the filtrate, concentrate to about 200ml.

(3) Add certain ethanol into the concentrated solution, and make the ethanol content 70%. Keep in cold storage and stand still above 24h.

(4) The ethanol in above solution was recycled after standing for above 24h. And the supernatant is heated and concentrated to about 70g after filtration.

(5) The fine powder of chlorphenamine is obtained by crushing and passing through No. 6 sieve, and then mix it well with the fine powder obtained in (1).

(6) Add the hot extract obtained in Step 4 into the mixture obtained in Step 5 to form a pasty mass. The mass is passed to make granules. The obtained granules are dried at 60~70℃ subsequently.

(7) Add 3% of talcum to the dry granules and mix well. Then compress into tablets.

Experiment flow chart (Figure 11-1):

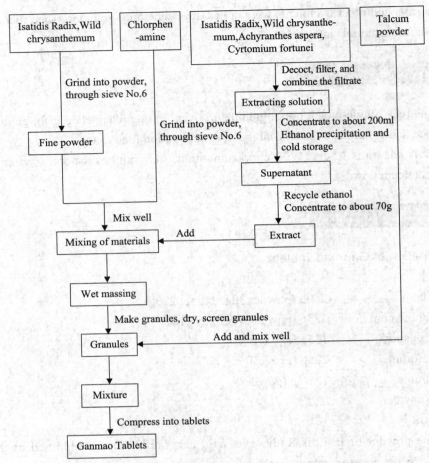

Figure 11-1　The preparation flow chart of Ganmao Tablets

【Characters】This product is brown semi-extract tablets, fragrant, bitter taste.

【Functions and Indications】Heat-clearing and detoxifying drugs. Used for early stage of a cold, cold and fever, headache and stuffy nose, sore throat, etc.

【Usage and Dosage】Oral, 4~6 tablets one time and 3 times one day.

【Considerations】The dosage proportion of extract material and powder material in the prescription of Chinese medicine semi-extract tablets could be adjusted according to the extract rate and powder yield of Chinese medicine.

(Ⅱ) Quality inspection of Ganmao Tablets

1. Characteristics Tables should have a complete and smooth appearance, and possess suitable hardness.

2. Weight variation Unless otherwise specified, the weight variation of the tablets should comply with the following requirement (Table 11-1).

Table 11-1　Weight variation limit for tablets products

Average weight or labeled weight	Weight variation limit
Less than 0.30g	±7.5%
0.30g or more than 0.30g	±5%

Inspection: Weight accurately 20 tablets and calculate the average weight, then weight individually each of the 20 tablets and compare the weight of each tablets with the average weight (if assay is not required, the weight of each tablets should be compared with the labeled weight). Not more than 2 of the individual tablets weights shall deviate from the average weight by more than the weight variation limit shown in table, and none deviate by twice the limit.

3. Disintegration　Unless otherwise specified, tablets should comply with the determination of disintegration (General rule 0921). The disintegration of the semi-extract tablets should occur no more than 60min.

4. Hardness　Unless otherwise specified, the hardness of tablets is determined by using a hardness tester, and the results should comply with the requirements.

5. Friability　The uncoated tablets should comply with the test for tablets friability (General rule 0923). Unless otherwise specified, the tablets should meet the requriments if no detected broken tablets, cracked or debris, and its weight loss is less than 1%.

Questions

1. Why should we prepare granules first before preparing tablets?

2. How to decide the dosage of extract material and powder material in the prescription of Chinese medicine semi-extract tablets?

3. Explain why and how to solve the problems if hardness, disintegration limit and weight variation are not qualified.

4. How to prevent the easy moisture absorption phenomenon of Chinese medicine extract tablets?

PPT

实验十二　胶囊剂的制备

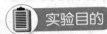 实验目的

1. **掌握**　硬胶囊剂的制备工艺过程及操作要点。
2. **熟悉**　硬胶囊剂的质量要求与质量检查方法。
3. **了解**　胶囊剂的分类及其特点。

实验提要

1. 胶囊剂系指将原料药物或与适宜辅料充填于空心胶囊或密封于软质囊材中制成的固体制剂。胶囊剂分为硬胶囊剂、软胶囊剂和肠溶胶囊剂。其特点包括：①外观整洁、美观、易吞服；②可掩盖药物的不良气味和减少药物的刺激性；③生物利用度高于片剂、丸剂等固体制剂；④可提高药物稳定性；⑤含液体或油量高的药物可制成软胶囊剂；⑥可将剂量小、难溶于水、胃肠道内不易吸收的药物溶于适当油中，制成软胶囊剂，利于药物吸收；⑦可延缓药物释放。

2. 空心胶囊以明胶为主要原料制成，近年来也有应用甲基纤维素、海藻酸钙、聚乙烯醇、变性明胶以及其他高分子材料，以改善胶囊剂的溶解度或产生肠溶性。硬质空胶囊呈圆筒形、质地坚硬、具有弹性，由上下配套的两节紧密套合而成。空胶囊规格共8种，规格越大，容积越小，常用0~5号。一般可先测定待填充物料的堆密度，然后根据应装剂量计算物料容积，以决定选用胶囊的号码。空胶囊规格及对应的容积见表12-1。

表 12-1　空胶囊规格及其容积对应表

空胶囊规格	000	00	0	1	2	3	4	5
容积（±10%）/ml	1.42	0.95	0.67	0.48	0.37	0.27	0.20	0.13

3. 制备工艺流程

（1）硬胶囊的制备工艺流程：空胶囊的制备 → 药物的处理 → 药物的填充 → 胶囊的封口 → 除粉和磨光 → 质检 → 包装。

（2）软胶囊的制备方法有压制法和滴制法两种。压制法（模压法）工艺流程：配制囊材胶液 → 制胶片 → 配制药液 → 压制 → 质检 → 包装。滴制法工艺流程：胶液和药液的配制 → 滴制 → 冷却 → 整丸 → 干燥 → 质检 → 包装。

（3）下列情况不宜制成胶囊剂：①药物的水溶液或乙醇溶液，因能使胶囊壁溶解；②易溶性药物如氯化钠、溴化物、碘化物等，以及小剂量的刺激性药物，因在胃中溶解后局部浓度过高而刺激胃黏膜；③易风化药物，因可使胶囊壁变软；④吸湿性药物，因可使胶囊壁过分干燥而变脆。

（4）硬胶囊中的药物，除特殊规定外，一般均要求是混合均匀的细粉或颗粒。以中药为原料的处方中剂量小的或细料药等，可直接粉碎成细粉，过六号筛，混匀后填充；剂量较大者可先

医药大学堂
WWW.YIYAO9XT.COM

将部分药材粉碎成细粉，其余药材提取浓缩成稠膏后与细粉混匀，干燥、研细、过筛、混匀后填充；也可将全部药材经提取浓缩成稠膏后加适当辅料制成细小颗粒，经干燥混匀后填充；如处方组成中含有结晶性或提取的纯品药物时，也应先研成细粉再与群药细粉混匀后填充。

实验器材

1. **仪器** 烧杯、烧瓶、40目筛、烘箱、分析天平、胶囊填充板或胶囊填充机、崩解仪等。

2. **试药** 金银花提取物、黄芩提取物、乙醇、淀粉。

实验操作步骤

（一）银黄胶囊

【处方】

金银花提取物	10g
黄芩提取物	4g
淀粉	16g
共制成 100 粒	

【制法】取金银花提取物、黄芩提取物、淀粉混匀，以75%乙醇溶液制软材，挤压过40目筛网制湿颗粒，40~50℃干燥，整粒，装胶囊，约制成100粒（每粒0.30g），即得。

银黄胶囊制备流程图如图12-1所示。

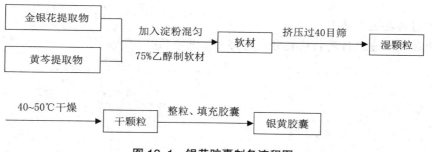

图 12-1 银黄胶囊制备流程图

【功能与主治】清热，解毒，消炎。用于急慢性扁桃体炎、急慢性咽喉炎、上呼吸道感染等症。

【用法与用量】口服，一次 2~4 粒，一日 4 次。

【规格】每粒装 0.3g 内容物。

【注意事项】

（1）黄芩中的主要有效成分为黄芩苷，提取时黄芩苷在一定温度下易被药材中的共存酶酶解成苷元而降低疗效，故提取时注意杀酶保苷，即直接用沸水提取，以使酶在高温下变性而避免其对黄芩苷的影响。

（2）金银花中的有效成分绿原酸对热不稳定，干燥过程中应严格控制温度，一般要求在60℃以下。

（3）硬胶囊剂中填充的药物，可以是混合均匀的细粉或颗粒。一般颗粒的流动性比细粉大，有利于胶囊剂的填充。若以颗粒填充，其粒度不宜过大，否则不易填充均匀，且填充量明显减少。一般以 30~40 目颗粒为宜。

（4）空胶囊规格常通过试装来确定。胶囊剂装量为 0.3~0.5g 时，可考虑选用 0~2 号空胶囊。

（5）装胶囊过程中应注意控制适当的温度和湿度。一般温度在 20~25℃，相对湿度在 30%~45%，以避免胶囊中的药粉或颗粒吸湿。

【附　金银花提取物、黄芩提取物的制备】

（1）**金银花提取物的制备**　取金银花分别加水 10 倍、7 倍煎煮 2 次，第一次 1 小时，第二次 45 分钟，滤过，滤液加入石灰乳调节 pH 至 10~12，静置，滤取沉淀，加适量水，加硫酸调节 pH 至 6~7，搅匀，滤过，滤液浓缩至稠膏状，烘干，即得。

（2）**黄芩提取物的制备**　取黄芩分别加水 8 倍、6 倍煎煮 2 次，每次 1 小时，合并煎液，滤过，滤液加硫酸调节 pH 至 2，静置，滤取沉淀，用乙醇适量洗涤后，干燥，即得。

（二）胶囊剂的质量检查

1. **性状**　本品为胶囊剂，内容物为黄棕色粉末；味微苦。

2. **水分**　胶囊剂按照水分测定法（通则 0832）检查，不得超过 9.0%。

3. **装量差异**　按照附录胶囊剂项下（通则 0103）方法检查，装量差异限度应在标示装量或平均装量的 ±10% 以内，超出装量差异限度的不得多于 2 粒，并不能有 1 粒超出限度 1 倍。

4. **崩解时限**　按照崩解时限检查法（通则 0921）检查，应在 30 分钟内全部崩解，如有 1 粒未能完全崩解，应另取 6 粒复试，均应符合规定。如有部分颗粒状物不能够通过筛网，但无硬心者，视为符合规定。

5. **其他**　应符合现行胶囊剂项下（通则 0103）有关的各项规定。

 思考题

1. 胶囊剂有哪些主要特点？

2. 制备中药硬胶囊进行药物填充时应有哪些注意事项？

题库

Experiment 12　Preparation of Capsules

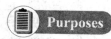

Purposes

1. To master the general process and the main operating points to produce capsules.
2. To be familiar with the quality requirements and quality control methods for capsules products.
3. To understand the main characteristics and classification of capsules.

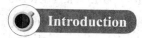

Introduction

1. Capsules are solid preparations by filling the APIs with suitable excipients into hollow capsule shells or soft capsules. Capsules can be divided into hard capsules, soft capsules and enteric capsules. The characteristics of capsule include: ① It should neat, attractive appearance and easy to swallow; ② It can mask the bad smell and reduce the irritation of drugs; ③ It may offer higher bioavailability than other solid preparations such as tablets and pills; ④ It may improve drug stability; ⑤ Drugs with high proportion of liquid or oil can be sealed into soft capsules; ⑥ Drugs with small dosage, poor dissolution in water, and low absorption in the gastrointestinal tract can be dissolved in appropriate oils and sealed into soft capsules to enhance the oral absorption; ⑦ Drugs can be sustained releasing from capsules.

2. The main material of hollow capsules is gelatin. In recent years, methylcellulose, calcium alginate, polyvinyl alcohol, denatured gelatin and other polymers have also been used to improve the solubility of the capsules or to produce enteric properties. The shell of hard capsule is cylindrical, hard in texture, and elastic. An entire hard capsule shell is made of two closely matched upper and lower parts. There are eight sizes of empty capsules. The larger the size, the smaller the capacity. No. 0 to 5 are common sizes. Generally, the bulk density of the content should be determined first, and then the volume of the material can be calculated according to the dosage to be filled to determine the number of the capsule could be selected according to the volume of the dosage of content . See the Table 12-1 for specifications of hollow shell of hard capsules and corresponding volumes.

Table 12-1　The size and capacity of hollow hard capsules

The size of capsule shell	000	00	0	1	2	3	4	5
Volume(±10%)/ml	1.42	0.95	0.67	0.48	0.37	0.27	0.20	0.13

3. Preparation procedures

(1) The procedure of hard capsules is: Preparation of capsule shells → drugs preparation→ fill capsules → seal capsules → powder removal and polishing → quality inspection → packaging.

(2) There are two methods for preparing soft capsules: compression method and dropping method. The procedure of pressing method is as follow: Preparation of capsule glue → film making → preparation of

medicinal solution→ pressing capsule → quality inspection → packaging. The process of dropping method is as follows: Preparation of glue solution and medicinal solution → dropping capsule → cooling → sorting → drying → quality inspection → packaging.

(3) The following cases are not suitable for capsules. ① The aqueous or ethanol solution of drugs, which can dissolve the capsule shell; ② Soluble drugs such as sodium chloride, bromide, iodide, etc., and irritant drugs with small dosage, of which the local concentration is too high to stimulate the gastric mucosa after dissolution in the stomach; ③ The easy to weather drugs, which can soft the capsule shell; ④ Hygroscopic drugs, which can make the capsule shell dry and brittle.

(4) Generally, drugs in hard capsules should be uniformly mixed fine powder or granules, unless otherwise specified. The small doses or fine medicines of TCM can be ground directly into fine powders, passed through a No. 6 sieve, mixed and then filled; larger doses parts can be ground into fine powders first, and the rest materials are extracted, concentrated into a thick paste and mixed with fine powder, dried, ground, sieved, and mixed then filled. All medicinal materials can also be extracted, concentrated into a thick paste and mixed with appropriate excipients to make fine particles. Then the particles are dried and mixed and filled. If the formulation contains crystalline or pure compounds, it should also be ground into fine powder and then mixed thoroughly with the other medicinal materials and filled.

 Equipments and Materials

1. Equipments　Beakers, flasks, 40 mesh pharmacopoeia sieve, oven, analytical balance, capsule filling plate or capsule filling machine, disintegration time tester.

2. Materials　Honeysuckle extract, Scutellaria baicalensis extract, ethanol, starch.

 Experimental Procedures

(Ⅰ) Preparation of Yinhuang Capsules

【Formula】

Honeysuckle extract	10g
Scutellaria baicalensis extract	4g
Starch	16g

Make into 100 capsules

【Preparation】 Take appropriate amount of honeysuckle extract, scutellaria baicalensis extract and starch, mix well with 75% ethanol solution to form a pasty mass. The mass is squeezed through a sieve of 40 mesh to make wet granules and then is dried at 40~50℃ followed by breaking and sorting the aggregated granules. The blended granules are filled into hollow capsules shell to about 100 capsules (0.30g / capsule).

The experimental procedure for the preparation of Yinhuang Capsules is shown in the Figure 12-1.

【Functions and Indications】 Heat-clearing, detoxifying and anti-inflammation drug. For acute and chronic tonsillitis, acute and chronic pharyngitis, upper respiratory tract infections and other symptoms.

【Usage and Dosage】 Orally, 2 to 4 capsules at one time, 4 times a day.

【Specifications】 0.3g of content per capsule.

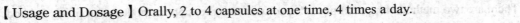

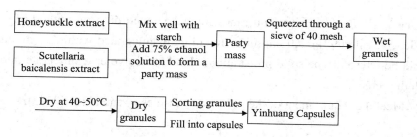

Figure 12-1   The Preparation procedure of Yinhuang Capsules

【Considerations】

(1) The main active ingredient in Scutellaria baicalensis is baicalin. At the time of extraction, baicalin is easily digested into baicalein by the coexisting enzymes in the medicinal materials and reduce the efficacy. Therefore, the boiling water should be used to denature the enzyme at high temperature and avoid the digestion effect on baicalin.

(2) The active ingredient chlorogenic acid in honeysuckle is unstable in heat. The dry temperature should be strictly controlled under 60℃.

(3) Hard capsules can be filled with drugs, which can be finely mixed powders or granules. Generally, the general granules show better fluidity than that of the fine powder and is beneficial to the capsules filling. If capsules are filled with granules, the particle size should not be too large, otherwise it is not easy to fill uniformly, and significantly reduces the filling amount. In generall, 30 to 40 mesh granules are suitable.

(4) The specifications of empty capsules are often determined by trial. When the capsule dosage is 0.3 ~ 0.5g, No. 0~2 hollow capsules shell can be considered.

(5) A proper temperature and humidity should be carefully controlled during capsule filling. The temperature is between 20 ~ 25℃ and the relative humidity is between 30% ~ 45%, so as to prevent the powder or granules in the capsule from absorbing moisture.

【Supplementary — the preparation of honeysuckle extract, scutellaria baicalensis extract】

(1) Preparation of honeysuckle extract: Take honeysuckle and decoct twice with 10 times and 7 times of water, 1 hour for the first time and 45 minutes for the second time. After filtration, the filtrate is added with lime milk to adjust the pH to 10 ~ 12. left to stand, filter and keep the precipitate. Add an appropriate amount of water. Add sulfuric acid to adjust the pH to 6 ~ 7. Mix well. Filter and concentrate the filtrate to the thick paste. Dry to obtain the final extracts.

(2) Preparation of Scutellaria baicalensis extract: Scutellaria baicalensis is decocted twice with 8 times and 6 times of water, 1 hour each time. The decoction was combined and filtered. The filtrate was adjusted to pH 2 with sulfuric acid, left to stand. Filter and keep the precipitate. Wash with appropriate amount of ethanol and dry to obtain the final extracts.

（Ⅱ） Quality Inspection of Yinhuang Capsules

1. Description   The content of capsules occurs as yellow-brown powder; taste slightly bitter.

2. Determination of water   Carry out the Determination of water (General rule 0832). The water should contain not more than 9.0 percent, unless otherwise specified.

3. Filling variation   The filling variation is checked according to the provision of capsules (General rule 0103). The variation should be within ± 10% of the marked or average weight. The amounts of capsules exceeding the limitation should not exceed two and no more than 1 capsule that exceeds the one

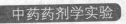

time of limitation.

4. Disintegration   The disintegration time is checked according to method of determination of disintegration (General rule 0921). All capsules should be disintegrated within 30 minutes. If one fails, another six should be retested. The solid preparations should dissolve or disintegrate into small particles and pass through the screen,

5. Others   Meet the requirement of the provision capsules (General rule 0103).

 Questions

1. What are the main characteristics of capsules?

2. What should be pay attention for drug filling step when preparing hard capsules for traditional Chinese medicine?

实验十三　膜剂的制备

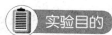 实验目的

1. **掌握**　膜剂的制备工艺过程及操作要点。
2. **熟悉**　膜剂成膜材料的种类与性能。
3. **了解**　膜剂的质量评价。

实验提要

1. 膜剂是指药物与适宜的成膜材料经加工制成的膜状剂型，供口服或黏膜用。膜剂的制备常采用涂膜法，即先将成膜材料制成溶浆，再加入药物混合均匀后涂膜，最后分割即可。

2. 常用的成膜材料多为水溶性高分子物质，包括天然的与合成的高分子材料。天然的成膜材料有淀粉、糊精、明胶、阿拉伯胶、白及胶、琼脂等；合成的成膜材料有聚乙烯醇（PVA）、乙烯－醋酸乙烯共聚物（EVA）、纤维素衍生物等。

3. 除成膜材料外，膜剂中常用的附加剂有：①增塑剂，如甘油、山梨醇等；②表面活性剂，如聚山梨酯 80、十二烷基硫酸钠等；③填充剂，如淀粉等；④着色剂与遮光剂，如色素、二氧化钛等；⑤矫味剂，如蔗糖等。

实验器材

1. **仪器**　烧杯、三角烧瓶、七号筛、烘箱、天平、恒温水浴锅、研钵、玻璃板。
2. **试药**　养阴生肌散、PVA（17-88）、甘油、聚山梨酯 80、75% 乙醇、85% 乙醇、液状石蜡、蒸馏水。

实验操作步骤

（一）养阴生肌膜的制备

【处方】

养阴生肌散	2g
PVA（17-88）	10g
甘油	1ml
聚山梨酯 80	5 滴
蒸馏水	50ml

【制法】取 PVA 加入 85% 乙醇浸泡过夜，滤过，沥干，重复处理 1 次，倾出乙醇，将 PVA 于 60℃ 烘干后，称取 10g，置于三角烧瓶中，加蒸馏水 50ml，水浴上加热，使之溶化成胶液。称取养阴生肌散（过七号筛）2g 于研钵中，加甘油 1ml，聚山梨酯 80 5 滴，研磨均匀，缓缓将

PVA 胶液加入，研匀，静置脱气泡后，供涂膜用。取出玻璃板（5cm×20cm）5 块，洗净，干燥，用 75% 乙醇涂擦消毒，再涂擦少许液状石蜡。用吸管吸取上述药液 10ml，滴注于玻璃板上，摊匀，水平晾至半干，于 60℃ 烘干，小心揭下药膜，即得。

实验流程图如图 13-1 所示。

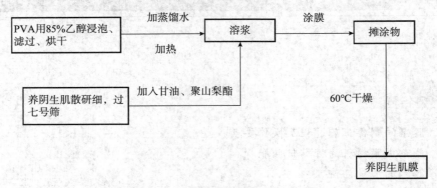

图 13-1　膜剂的制备工艺流程图

【性状】本品为无气泡的绿色药膜。

【功能与主治】清热解毒。用于湿热性口腔溃疡、复发性口腔溃疡及疱疹性口腔炎。

【用法与用量】取适量贴于口腔患处。

【注意事项】PVA 溶解后应趁热过滤，以除去杂质，以免放冷后不易过滤；药物与胶浆混匀后应静置除去气泡，涂膜时不宜搅拌，以免形成气泡。

（二）膜剂的质量检查

1. **外观**　膜剂外观应完整光洁，厚度一致，色泽均匀，无明显气泡。

2. **重量差异**　按照 2020 年版《中国药典》总则中膜剂项下方法检查，装量差异限度应满足表 13-1 的要求，超出重量差异限度的不得多于 2 片，并不能有 1 片超出限度 1 倍。凡检查了含量均匀度的膜剂，一般不再进行重量差异检查。

表 13-1　膜剂的重量差异限度规定

平均重量	重量差异限度
0.02g 及 0.02g 以下	±15%
0.02g 以上至 0.20g	±10%
0.20g 以上	7.5%

 思考题

1. 处方中聚乙烯醇、甘油、聚山梨酯 80、蒸馏水各有何作用？

2. 制备膜剂的操作要点有哪些？

题库

Experiment 13　Preparation of Pellicles

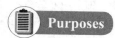
Purposes

1. To master the preparation methods and key operations of pellicles.
2. To be familiar with the types and properties of film-forming materials of pellicles.
3. To understand the quality inspection methods of pellicles.

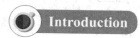
Introduction

1. Pellicles are preparations of pellicular form processed by the drug substances with appropriate pellicular materials. They are intended for oral use or topical use on external mucous membranes. Solvent-casting method is ideal for manufacturing pellicles, that the dry ingredients for the pellicle are heated until they are molten, blend the drug into it uniformly for filming, and then cut up the film.

2. Water-soluble polymer materials are the most commonly used film-forming materials, including natural and synthetic polymer materials. The natural materials include starch, dextrin, gelatin, acacia, bletilla colloid, and agar, etc; PVA, EVA and cellulose derivative are the synthetic film-forming materials.

3. Plasticizers such as glycerol and sorbitol, surfactants such as polysorbate 80 and sodium dodecyl sulfate, filler such as starch, colorant such as pigment, sunscreen such as titanium dioxide and flavoring such as sucrose are commonly used as additional agents for the preparation of pellicles except the film-forming materials.

Equipments and Materials

1. Equipments　Beaker, conical flask, No.7 sieve, oven, balance, thermostat water bath, mortar, glass plate, etc.

2. Materials　Yangyin Shengji powder, PVA(17-88), glycerol, polysorbate 80, 75% ethanol, 85% ethanol, liquid paraffin, distilled water, etc.

Experimental Procedures

（Ⅰ）Preparation of Yangyin Shengji Pellicle

【Formula】

Yangyin Shengji powder	2g
PVA(17-88)	10g
Glycerol	1ml
Polysorbate 80	5 drops

Distilled water   50ml

【Preparation】Add 85% ethanol into PVA, soak overnight, filter, drain and repeat again. Dry PVA in the oven of 60℃ after pouring the ethanol out. Put 10g the processed PVA in the bottle, add 50ml distilled water and heat it on a water bath until the mixture totally dissolves. Put 2g Yangyin Shengji powder(sieved through the 7 mesh sieve) in a mortar, add 1ml glycerol and polysorbate 80 and dispersed evenly by constant grinding. Transfer PVA solution into the mixture in a steady stream, grind them uniformly and remove air bubbles by standing for a while for filming. Wash 5 glass plates(5cm×20cm), apply 75% ethanol on them to sterilize after dried, and apply a little liquid paraffin on them. Suck 10ml mixture with a dropper, drop it on the glass plates, spread the mixture out, dry in the air and in the oven under 60℃, and detach the film.

Experiment flow chart (Figure 13-1):

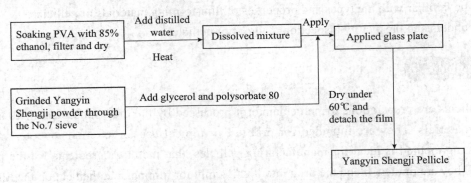

Figure 13-1   Preparation procedure of pellicles

【Characters】This product is a green medicine film without bubbles.

【Functions and Indications】Clear heat and detoxificate for damp-heat oral ulcer, recurrent oral ulcer and herpes stomatitis.

【Usage and Dosage】Put proper amount and stick it to the affected part in the mouth.

【Considerations】After the PVA is dissolved, it should be filtered while hot to remove impurities, because it is not easy to filter after cooling. After mixing the drug with PVA solution, it should be kept still to remove the air bubbles. It is not suitable to stir when applying the film to avoid the appearance of air bubbles.

(Ⅱ) Quality Inspection of Yangyin Shengji Pellicle

1. Appearance   The pellicle should be complete and smooth, consistent thickness, uniform color and no obvious bubbles.

2. Weight variation   The weight variation should comply with the following requirements which are listed in the Table 13-1 according to the *Chineses Pharmacopoeia*. Not more than 2 samples should deviate from the average weight by the limit of weight variation, and none should deviate by more than twice of the limit. Where the test for content uniformity is specified, the test for weight variation may not be required.

Table 13-1   Requirements of weight variation of pellicles

Average weight	Limit of weight variation
0.02g or less	±15%
More than 0.02g to 0.20g	±10%
More than 0.20g	7.5%

Questions

1. What is the effect of PVA, glycerol, polysorbate 80 and distilled water in the formula?
2. What is the key points of the preparation of Yangyin Shengji Pellicle?

实验十四　灸剂的制备

PPT

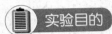　**实验目的**

熟悉　中药灸剂的制备方法、关键操作和注意事项。

实验提要

1. 灸剂是将艾叶捣、碾成绒状，或另加其他药料卷制成卷烟状或捻成其他形状，供熏灼穴位或其他患部的以预防或治疗疾病为目的的外用制剂。

2. 艾绒的制备方法：取艾叶的干燥品，筛去灰屑及杂质，置石臼或其他粉碎装置中粉碎成棉绒状，拣去叶脉，即得。

3. 药艾条是《中国药典》收录的一种灸剂。其主要成分为艾叶，艾叶为菊科植物艾 *Artemisia argyi* Lévl. et Vant. 的干燥叶，含挥发性成分。

实验器材

1. **仪器**　粉碎机、药筛、低温干燥机。

2. **试药**　艾叶、桂枝、高良姜、广藿香、降香、香附、白芷、陈皮、丹参、生川乌、白棉纸（28cm×15cm）、胶水。

实验操作步骤

灸剂的制备
药艾条
【处方】

艾叶	40g
桂枝	2.5g
高良姜	2.5g
广藿香	1g
降香	3.5g
香附	1g
白芷	2g
陈皮	1g
丹参	1g
生川乌	1.5g

【制法】以上十味，艾叶碾成艾绒；其余桂枝等九味粉碎成细粉，过筛，混匀。取艾绒 20g，均匀平铺在一张长 28cm，宽 15cm 的白棉纸上，再均匀撒布上述粉末 8g，将棉纸两端折叠约6cm，卷紧成条，粘合封闭，低温干燥，即得。

实验流程图如图 14-1 所示。

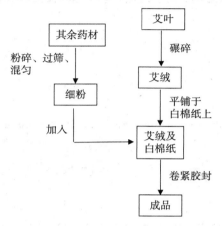

图 14-1　灸剂的制备工艺流程图

【性状】本品呈圆柱状，长 20~21cm，直径 1.7~1.8cm；气香，点燃后不熄灭，烟气特异。

【功能与主治】行气血，逐寒湿。用于风寒湿痹，肌肉酸麻，关节四肢疼痛，脘腹冷痛。

【用法与用量】直射灸法，一次适量，红晕为度，一日 1~2 次；或遵医嘱。

【规格】每支重 28g。

【贮藏】密闭，防潮。

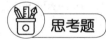 **思考题**

在制备过程中，为什么要采取低温干燥？

题库

Experiment 14　Preparation of Moxibustion Formula

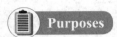 **Purposes**

To be familiar with the preparation methods, key operations and matters needing attention of Chinese herbal moxibustion formula.

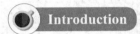 **Introduction**

1. Moxibustion formula is a kind of external preparation for the purpose of prevention or treatment of diseases, which is made from artemisiae argyi folium crushed into fluffy state, or added with other medicine materials which are rolled into cigarette shape or twisted into other shapes for fumigating acupoints or other affected parts.

2. Preparation of moxa floss: Take dry products of artemisiae argyi folium, screen ash crumbs and impurities, crush them into cotton velvet state in stone mortar or other crushing device, pick out leaf veins.

3. Yao'aitiao is a kind of moxibustion formula collected in the *Chinese Pharmacopoeia*. Its main component is the artemisiae argyi folium, dried leaves of *Artemisiae Argyi* Lévl. et Vant. from asteraceae, containing volatile ingredients.

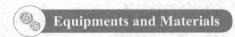 **Equipments and Materials**

1. Equipments　Grinding mill, medical sieve, low-temperature drier.

2. Materials　Artemisiae Argyi Folium, Cinnamomi Ramulus, Alpiniae Offic-inarum Rhizoma, Pogostemonis Herba, Dalbergiae Odoriferae Lignum, Cyperi Rhizoma, Angelicae Dahuricae Radix, Citri Reticulatae Pericarpium, Salviae Mi-ltiorrhizae Radix Et Rhizoma, Aconiti Radix(not prepared), white cotton-paper (28cm×15cm), gluewater.

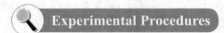 **Experimental Procedures**

Preparation of Moxibustion Formula

Yao'aitiao

【Formula】

Artemisiae Argyi Folium	40g
Cinnamomi Ramulus	2.5g
Alpiniae Officinarum Rhizoma	2.5g
Pogostemonis Herba	1g

Dalbergiae Odoriferae Lignum	3.5g
Cyperi Rhizoma	1g
Angelicae Dahuricae Radix	2g
Citri Reticulatae Pericarpium	1g
Salviae Miltiorrhizae Radix Et Rhizoma	1g
Aconiti Radix	1.5g

【Preparation】Artemisiae argyi folium are crushed into moxa floss. Pulverize all the other ingredients to fine powders, sift and mix completely. Spread 20g of the moxa floss on a sheet of white cotton-paper of 28cm in length and 15cm in width and scatter evenly 8g of the above powder on it. Fold the two ends of the paper about 6cm, roll it tightly into strips and dry it at a low temperature after the process of gluing and sealing.

Experiment flow chart (Figure 14-1):

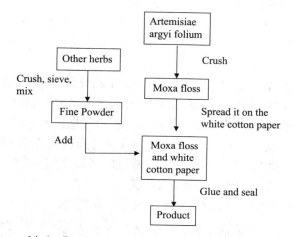

Figure 14-1　Preparation procedure of moxibustion formula

【Characters】The product is cylindrical, 20~21cm long and 1.7~1.8cm in diameter. A smoke that emits a specific smell after ignition doesn't go out easily after being ignited.

【Functions and Indications】Contribute to the appropriate flow of qi and blood, and expel coldness and dampness. Used for wind-cold-dampness arthralgia, muscle soreness and numbness, pain in joints and limbs, cold and pain in abdomen.

【Usage and Dosage】To be applied for direct moxibustion until the appearance of glow. 1~2 times a day or follow the advice of physician .

【Specifications】Each weighs 28g.

【Storage】Hermetic seal, moisture proof.

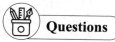 **Questions**

Why should low temperature drying be adopted in the preparation process?

PPT

实验十五　β- 环糊精包合物的制备

实验目的

1. **掌握**　饱和水溶液法制备包合物的工艺及操作要点。
2. **熟悉**　β- 环糊精包合物的性质及应用。
3. **了解**　其他主分子的性质及应用。

实验提要

1. 包合物是由主分子和客分子两部分组成，主分子具有较大的空穴结构，能将客分子容纳在内形成分子囊。包合技术的优点如下：增加药物的稳定性，增加药物的溶解度，掩盖不良气味，减少药物的刺激性，调节药物的释药速率，使液体药物粉末化，提高药物生物利用度。

2. 环糊精是由多个 D- 葡萄糖分子以 α-（1，4）糖苷键连接的环状低聚糖化合物，为环状中空圆筒形结构，具有疏水的内部和亲水的外部。常见的环糊精有 α、β、γ 三种，分别由 6、7、8 个葡萄糖分子构成，其中以 β- 环糊精应用最为广泛。

3. 环糊精包合物制备方法较多，有饱和水溶液法、研磨法、冷冻干燥法、喷雾干燥法等，可根据环糊精和药物的性质，结合实际生产条件加以选用。本实验采用饱和水溶液法，先配制环糊精饱和溶液，在搅拌下加入一定比例的药物，搅拌直到成为包合物。

实验器材

1. **仪器**　具塞锥形瓶、恒温水浴锅、电子天平、冰箱、干燥器、布氏漏斗等。
2. **试药**　β- 环糊精、薄荷油、无水乙醇、蒸馏水。

实验操作步骤

（一）薄荷油 –β– 环糊精包合物的制备

【处方】

β- 环糊精	4g
薄荷油	1ml
蒸馏水	50ml

【制法】取 100ml 具塞锥形瓶，称取 4g β- 环糊精置于 50ml 蒸馏水中，加热溶解。降温至 50℃，滴加薄荷油 1ml，恒温搅拌 2.5 小时。冷藏 24 小时，待沉淀完全后，滤过。用无水乙醇洗涤沉淀 3 次，每次 5ml，至沉淀表面近无油渍，将包合物置于干燥器中干燥，即得。

医药大学堂
WWW.YIYAODXT.COM

实验流程图如图 15-1 所示。

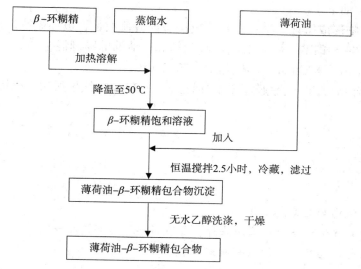

图 15-1 $\beta-$ 环糊精包合物的制备工艺流程图

【性状】 本品为有特殊气味的白色粉末。

【注意事项】

（1）薄荷油主要成分为薄荷脑、薄荷酮等，具有发汗、抗菌、解痉等作用。薄荷油容易挥发，制成环糊精包合物后可减少薄荷油挥发。药物的加入方法有 3 种：水溶性药物，直接加至环糊精的饱和溶液中，搅拌，制成包合物；水难溶性固体药物，可先溶于少量丙酮或异丙醇等有机溶剂中，再加至环糊精的饱和溶液中；水难溶性液体药物（如挥发油），直接加至环糊精的饱和溶液中，经搅拌至包合物完全形成。

（2）饱和水溶液法包合过程中，影响包合工艺的主要因素有主客分子投料比例、包合温度、包合时间、搅拌方式等。其中投料比和包合温度最为重要，投料比一般在 1∶3~1∶10（油∶$\beta-$ 环糊精，ml/g）的范围内，环糊精在水中的溶解度见表 15-1。

表 15-1 不同温度下环糊精在水中的溶解度（mg/g）

$t/℃$	α-CD	β-CD	γ-CD	$t/℃$	α-CD	β-CD	γ-CD
20	90	16.4	185	45	285	44	585
25	127	18.8	256	50	347	52.7	
30	165	22.8	320	60		72.9	
35	204	28.3	390	70		120.3	
40	242	34.9	460	80		196.6	

包合温度一般定在 30~60℃较适宜，增加包合温度可提高包合率，但包合温度过高也会影响药物的稳定性，如果药物是挥发油，会使挥发速度加快。

（二）$\beta-$ 环糊精包合物的质量检查

1. 包合率测定 取 $\beta-$ 环糊精包合物 3g，置 250ml 圆底烧瓶中加水 150ml，用挥发油提取器提取挥发油，参照《中国药典》挥发油测定法测定挥发油，按下式计算包合率。

$$包合率（\%）= \frac{W_4 \times W_1}{W_3 \times W_2} \times 100\%$$

式中，W_1 为 β- 环糊精包合物总量（g）；W_2 为测定时取样量（g）；W_3 为包合时用的挥发油总量（g）；W_4 为测得挥发油量（g）。

2. 环糊精包合物形成验证 采用差热分析法验证薄荷油是否被环糊精包入空穴。测试样品：β- 环糊精包合物、β- 环糊精、薄荷油、β- 环糊精和薄荷油的物理混合物。差热分析条件：参比物，α-Al$_2$O$_3$；升温速率，8℃/min；温度范围，20~340℃。

验证环糊精包合物形成的方法除差热分析法外，还有 X 射线衍射法、电镜扫描法、红外可见分光光度法等。

题库

📝 思考题

1. 本实验中应注意哪些关键操作？
2. 制备包合物的方法除饱和水溶液法外，还有哪些？各有何特点？
3. 使用环糊精包合物在药剂学上有何意义？

Experiment 15 Preparation of β-cyclodextrin Inclusion Compound

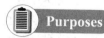
Purposes

1. To master the process and operation of saturated water solution method to prepare the inclusion compound.

2. To be familiar with the properties and applications of β-cyclodextrin.

3. To understand the properties and applications of the other host molecules.

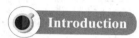
Introduction

1. Inclusion compound is composed by guest molecule and host molecule, the host molecule have major cavity structure that can contain guest molecule to form molecular capsules. The advantages of inclusion technique are: increase the stability of the drug, enhance solubility of the drug, mask unpleasant taste and reduce irritation of the drug, modify release profile of the drug, make liquid drug powdered, enhance bioavailability of poorly soluble drugs.

2. Cyclodextrins(CDs) are cyclic oligosaccharide compounds linked by a plurality of D-glucose molecules with α-(1,4) glycosidic linkages with a cyclic hollow cylindrical structure. CDs are molecular capsules with a hydrophobic inside and a hydrophilic outside. There are generally three types of CDs, α-CD, β-CD and γ-CD, which are made up of 6, 7, 8 D-glucose, respectively, and β-CD is most frequently used in inclusion technique.

3. The cyclodextrin inclusion compounds are prepared by different methods, such as saturated water solution method, grinding method, freeze-dry method, spray-dry method, and so on, which was selected by the cyclodextrin properties, drug properties and practical production conditions. The saturated water solution method is most frequently used: firstly prepare CD saturated solution, then add a certain percentage of the drug under stirring, until it becomes inclusion compound.

Equipments and Materials

1. Equipments Conical flask with stopper, thermostat water bath, analytical balance, refrigerator, desiccator, Buchner funnel, etc.

2. Materials β-cyclodextrin, peppermint oil, absolute ethyl alcohol, distilled water.

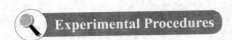 **Experimental Procedures**

（Ⅰ）Preparation of Peppermint Oil β−CD Inclusion Complex

【Formula】

β−CD	4g
Peppermint Oil	1ml
Distilled water	50ml

【Preparation】Add 4g of β−CD in 50ml distilled water in a 100ml conical flask with stopper, heat to dissolve β−CD. Allow to cool to 50℃, add 1ml of peppermint oil, stir for 2.5 hour at 50℃. Cool down for 24 hour in refrigerator, filter and wash the precipitate with absolute ethyl alcohol (each 5ml) for three times to the oil stains on the surface of precipitate disappeared, dry and store the product in a desiccator.

Experiment flow chart (Figure 15−1):

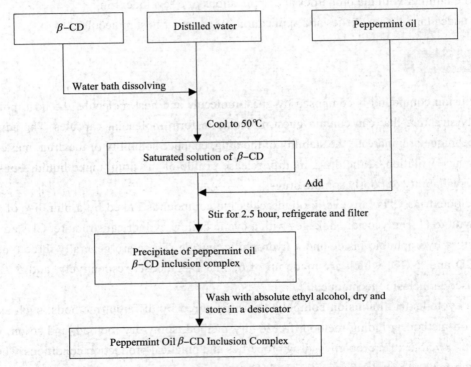

Figure 15−1   Preparation procedure of β−cyclodextrin Inclusion Compound

【Characters】This product is white powder with a special smell.

【Considerations】

(1) Peppermint Oil is an herbal supplement, mainly composed of menthol and menthol ketone, that has found to be effective as treatment for common cold, indigestion, inflammation of mouth/pharynx, irritable bowel syndrome, nausea, vomiting. Peppermint oil is a volatile compound that can be protected from evaporation by inclusion. There are three ways to add drugs: Water-soluble drugs can be directly added in the saturated solution of β−CD, and then the solution is stirred to prepare the inclusion compound. Water-insoluble solid drugs can be dissolved in a small amount of organic solvents (acetone or isopropanol), and then added in the saturated solution of β−CD. Water-insoluble liquid drugs, such as volatile oils, can be directly added in the saturated solution of β−CD, and then the solution is stirred to

prepare the inclusion compound.

(2) To prepare the inclusion compound by saturated water solution method, the main factors influencing the inclusion rate depends on the ratio of β–CD and drug, operating temperature, operating time and stirring modes, especially raw ratio and operating temperature. The ratio of β–CD and drug is considered to be optimal about $1:3\sim1:10$ oil: β–CD, ml/g. The solubility of cyclodextrin in water is shown in the Table 15–1.

Table 15–1   The solubility of cyclodextrin in water at different temperatures (mg/g)

$t/°C$	α–CD	β–CD	γ–CD	$t/°C$	α–CD	β–CD	γ–CD
20	90	16.4	185	45	285	44	585
25	127	18.8	256	50	347	52.7	
30	165	22.8	320	60		72.9	
35	204	28.3	390	70		120.3	
40	242	34.9	460	80		196.6	

The operating temperature is considered to be optimal about $30\sim60°C$. The inclusion rate can be increased by increasing the operating temperature. On the other hand, the stability of the drug is also affected by the too high operating temperature. For example, too high operating temperature would speed up the volatilization of volatile oils.

(II) Quality Inspection of Inclusion Compound

1. Determination of inclusion rate   Add 3g of the product to 150ml of water in a flask (250ml), extract the volatile oil with a set of steam distillation apparatus in accordance with ChP Appendix. The inclusion rate is calculated as follows:

$$\text{Inclusion rate}(\%) = \frac{W_4 \times W_1}{W_3 \times W_2} \times 100\%$$

Where, W_1 is the weight of total products (g); W_2 is the weight of tested products (g); W_3 is the weight of volatile oil used totally (g); W_4: weight of volatile oil extracted from the tested products (g).

2. Evaluation of cyclodextrin inclusion compounds   The evaluation of cyclodextrin inclusion compounds is to identify whether the peppermint oil is included into cyclodextrin by differential scanning calorimetry (DSC). The thermal behavior is studied by heating samples (inclusion compound, β–CD, peppermint oil, the physical mixture of β–CD and peppermint oil)at a rate of 8°C/min from 20 to 340°C. α–Al$_2$O$_3$ is used as the reference substance.

In addition to differential scanning calorimetry, X–ray diffraction, scanning electron microscopy and infrared visible spectrophotometry were used to evaluate the cyclodextrin inclusion compounds.

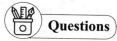 **Questions**

1. What are the keys to the preparation of cyclodextrin inclusion compound?

2. Are there other methods can be used to prepare the inclusion compound? Describe the advantages and disadvantages of these methods.

3. What is significance of the preparation of inclusuion compound in pharmacy?

实验十六 脂质体的制备

 实验目的

1. **掌握** 脂质体的制备方法、操作关键和注意事项。
2. **熟悉** 用阳离子交换树脂法测定脂质体包封率的方法。
3. **了解** 脂质体的形成原理、作用特点。

实验提要

1. 脂质体系指一种人工细胞膜，它具有封闭的球形结构，可使药物被保护在它的结构中，发挥定向作用。脂质体系指将药物包封于类脂双分子层形成的薄膜中所制成的超微型球状囊泡。根据类脂双分子层的层数，脂质体可分为单室脂质体（含大、小单室）和多室脂质体。特别适于作为抗癌药物载体，以改善药物的治疗作用，降低毒副作用等。

2. 制备脂质体的材料主要有磷脂和胆固醇。磷脂有天然磷脂（豆磷脂、卵磷脂等）和合成磷脂（二棕榈酰磷脂酰胆碱、二硬脂酰磷脂酰胆碱等）。胆固醇为两亲性物质，与磷脂混合使用，其作用是调节双分子层的流动性，减低脂质体膜的通透性。其他附加剂如十八胺、磷脂酸等，具有改变脂质体表面电荷的作用。

3. 脂质体的制法有多种，应根据药物的性质或用药需要进行选择。经典的薄膜分散法可形成多室脂质体，经超声处理后可得到小单室脂质体。此法操作简便，但包封率较低。

（1）**注入法** 有乙醚注入法和乙醇注入法两种，前者是将磷脂等溶于乙醚中，在搅拌下慢慢滴于55~65℃含药或不含药的水性介质中，蒸去乙醚，继续搅拌1~2小时，即可形成脂质体。

（2）**薄膜分散法** 将磷脂、胆固醇等类脂质及脂溶性药物溶于三氯甲烷（或其他有机溶剂）中，然后将三氯甲烷溶液在烧瓶中旋转蒸发，使其在内壁上形成薄膜后，加入含有水溶性药物的缓冲溶液，进行振摇，则可形成多室脂质体。

（3）**反相蒸发法** 将磷脂等脂溶性成分溶于有机溶剂（如三氯甲烷等）中，再与含药的缓冲液混合、乳化，然后减压蒸去有机溶剂而形成脂质体，适合于水溶性大分子活性物质，包封率高。

（4）**冷冻干燥法** 适于水中不稳定药物脂质体的制备。

（5）**熔融法** 制备的脂质体为多相脂质体，其性质稳定，可加热灭菌。

4. 包封率是评价脂质体内在质量的一个重要指标，常见的包封率测定方法有分子筛法、超速离心法、超滤膜法和阳离子交换树脂法等。

 实验器材

1. **仪器** 烧杯、天平、磁力搅拌器、显微镜。
2. **试药** 盐酸小檗碱、豆磷脂、胆固醇、乙醚、磷酸氢二钠、磷酸二氢钠、蒸馏水。

💬 **实验操作步骤**

（一）脂质体的制备

盐酸小檗碱脂质体

【处方】

盐酸小檗碱溶液（1mg·ml^{-1}）	25ml
豆磷脂	0.75g
胆固醇	0.25g
乙醚	35ml

共制成脂质体 25ml

【制法】

（1）磷酸盐缓冲液（PBS）的配制　称取磷酸氢二钠（Na$_2$HPO$_4$·12H$_2$O）3.7g 与磷酸二氢钠（NaH$_2$PO$_4$·2H$_2$O）20g，加蒸馏水适量，加热溶解，稀释成 1000ml，即得 0.067mol·L^{-1} 的磷酸盐缓冲液（pH 约为 5.7）。

（2）盐酸小檗碱溶液的配制　称取盐酸小檗碱适量，用 0.067mol·L^{-1} 磷酸盐缓冲液配成 1mg·ml^{-1} 的药液。

（3）盐酸小檗碱脂质体的制备　称取处方量豆磷脂、胆固醇置 150ml 小烧杯中，加入 35ml 乙醚，在磁力搅拌器上搅拌溶解，加入盐酸小檗碱溶液 25ml（1mg·ml^{-1}），继续搅拌，乳化，直到乙醚挥尽成为黄色的乳状液，即为小檗碱脂质体。

实验流程图如图 16-1 所示。

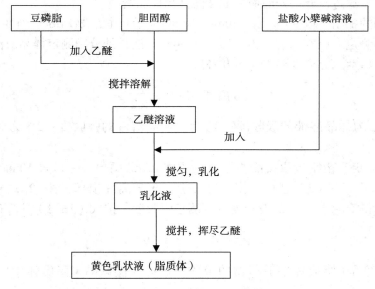

图 16-1　脂质体的制备工艺流程图

【性状】 本品为均匀的黄色乳状液。

【注意事项】

（1）注入法实验过程中，温度可控制在 50~60℃，操作中始终伴随搅拌，加入盐酸小檗碱溶液后搅拌的时间不得少于 2 小时。因脂质体形成有个过程，温度、滴加速度和搅拌时间对脂质体的形成均有影响。

（2）溶解磷脂和胆固醇的乙醚溶液应澄清，否则需过滤除去杂质。

（3）脂质体的粒径直接影响到其在体内的分布，因此，必须保证脂质体在贮存期间粒径不发生变化。可采用以下两种方法：①增加脂质体的ζ电位，ζ电位越大说明脂质体表面所带电荷越多，相互之间的静电斥力也越大，使脂质体不易凝集，增加脂质体的稳定性，因此，制备脂质体时，加入带电荷的脂质成分可使粒径变化减少到最低程度。②采用冷冻干燥的方法可以提高脂质体的物理和化学稳定性。

（二）盐酸小檗碱脂质体包封率的测定

1. 阳离子交换树脂分离柱的制备　称取已处理好的阳离子交换树脂约 1.5g，装于底部已垫有少量玻璃棉的 5ml 注射器筒中，加入 PBS 水化阳离子交换树脂，自然滴尽 PBS，即得。

2. 柱分离度考察

（1）空白脂质体的制备　称取豆磷脂 0.9g、胆固醇 0.3g 于小烧杯中，加乙醚 10ml，搅拌使溶解，旋转该小烧杯使乙醚液在杯壁成膜，用吸耳球吹风，将乙醚挥去。另取磷酸盐缓冲液 30ml 于小烧杯中，置磁力搅拌器上，加热至 55~65℃ 备用。取预热的磷酸盐缓冲液 20ml 加至含有磷脂和胆固醇成膜的小烧杯中，再将小烧杯置磁力搅拌器上，于 55~60℃ 保温 10 分钟，再在同样的温度下，搅拌 30~60 分钟（溶液体积减少，补加 PBS），即得。

（2）盐酸小檗碱与空白脂质体混合液的制备　精密量取 3mg·ml⁻¹ 的盐酸小檗碱溶液 0.1ml，置小试管中，加入 0.2ml 空白脂质体，混匀，即得。

（3）对照品溶液的制备　取盐酸小檗碱与空白脂质体混合液 0.1ml 置 10ml 量瓶中，加入 95% 乙醇 6ml，振摇使之溶解，再加 PBS 至刻度，摇匀，即得。

（4）样品溶液的制备　取盐酸小檗碱与空白脂质体混合液 0.1ml 加至分离柱顶部，待柱顶部的液体消失后，放置 5 分钟，仔细加入 PBS（注意不能将柱顶部离子交换树脂冲散），进行洗脱（需 1.5~2ml PBS），同时收集洗脱液于 10ml 量瓶中，加入 95% 乙醇 6ml 振摇使之溶解，再加 PBS 至刻度，摇匀，滤过，弃去初滤液，取续滤液为样品溶液。

（5）空白溶剂的配制　取 95% 乙醇 30ml，置 50ml 量瓶中，加 PBS 至刻度，摇匀，即得。

（6）吸收度的测定　以空白溶剂为对照，在 345nm 波长处分别测定样品溶液与对照品溶液的吸收度，计算柱分离度。分离度要求大于 0.95。

$$柱分离度 = 1 - \frac{A_样}{A_对 \times 2.5} \qquad （16-1）$$

式（16-1）中，$A_样$ 为样品溶液的吸收度；$A_对$ 为对照品溶液的吸收度；2.5 为对照品溶液的稀释倍数。

3. 供试品的测定　精密量取盐酸小檗碱脂质体 0.1ml 两份，一份置 10ml 量瓶中，按"2. 柱分离度考察"项下（2）~（3）进行操作；另一份置于分离柱顶部，按"2. 柱分离度考察"项下（4）进行操作，所得溶液于 345nm 波长处分别测定吸收度，按式（16-2）计算包封率。

$$包封率 = \frac{A_L}{A_r} \times 100\% \qquad （16-2）$$

式中，A_L 为柱分离后（脂质体中）药物的吸收度；A_r 为供试品（脂质体中、外）药物总的吸收度。

（三）脂质体的质量检查

1. 粒径与形态　用显微镜观察脂质体的粒径大小与形态，为多层囊状或多层圆球，大部分粒径在 0.7~1.2μm 之间。

2. 包封率的测定　测定脂质体中的总药量后，借用适当的方法分离脂质体，分别测定脂质体中包封的药量和介质中未包封的药量，按公式（16-3）和（16-4）计算包封率。

$$包封率 = \frac{药物总量 - 介质中未包封的药量}{药物总量} \times 100\% \qquad （16-3）$$

$$包封率 = \frac{脂质体中包封的药量}{脂质体中包封的药量 + 介质中未包封的药量} \times 100\% \qquad (16-4)$$

3. 渗漏率 根据给药途径的不同，将脂质体分散贮存在一定介质中，保持一定温度，于不同时间进行分离处理，测定介质中的药量，与贮存前包封的药量比较，按式（16-5）计算渗漏率。

$$渗漏率 = \frac{贮存后渗漏到介质中的药量}{贮存前包封的药量} \times 100\% \qquad (16-5)$$

4. 有机溶剂残留量 按照《中国药典》（2020 年版）总则中残留溶剂测定法，测定脂质体中有机溶剂残留量，应符合规定。

思考题

1. 制备脂质体时加入胆固醇的目的是什么？
2. 基质中加入药物时，注意事项是什么？
3. 注入法制备脂质体的关键是什么？
4. 脂质体作为抗癌药物载体的机制和特点有哪些？

题库

Experiment 16 Preparation of Liposomes

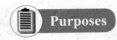

Purposes

1. To master the preparation methods, key operations and precautions of liposomes.

2. To be familiar with the method of cation exchange resin to determine the entrapment efficiency of liposomes.

3. To understand the formation mechanison and action characteristics of liposomes.

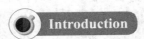

Introduction

1. Liposomes are dosed spherical vesides composed of artifical all membranes, which allow drugs to be protected in its structure and play a targeted role. Liposomes are ultra-micro spherical carrier made by encapsulating drugs in a film formed by a lipid bilayer. According to the number of lipid bilayers, liposomes can be divided into single-compartment liposomes (including large and small single-compartment liposomes) and multi-compartment liposomes. It is especially suitable as an anti-cancer drug carrier to improve the therapeutic effect of the drug and reduce toxic and side effects.

2. The materials used to make liposomes are mainly phospholipids and cholesterol. Phospholipids include natural phospholipids (soybean phospholipid, lecithin, etc.) and synthetic phospholipids (dipalmit oylphosphatidylcholine, distearylphosphatylcholine, etc.). Cholesterol is an amphiphilic substance, mixed with phospholipids, and its role is to regulate the fluidity of the bilayer and reduce the permeability of the liposome membrane. Other additives, such as stearylamine, phosphatidic acid, etc., have the property of changing the surface charge of liposomes.

3. There are many ways to make liposomes, which should be selected according to the nature of the drug or the needs of the drug. The classic thin-film dispersion method can form multi-compartment liposomes, and small-compartment liposomes can be obtained after ultrasonic treatment. This method is easy to operate, but the encapsulation rate is low.

(1) Injection method There are two methods: ether injection method and ethanol injection method. The former is to dissolve phospholipids in ether, and slowly drop it into the drug-containing or drug-free aqueous medium under stirring at 55~65°C. Evaporate the ether. Continue stirring for 1~2h, liposome is formed.

(2) Film dispersion method The lipid and lipid soluble drugs such as phospholipid and cholesterol are dissolved in chloroform (or other organic solvents), and then the chloroform solution is rotated and evaporated in a flask to form a film on the inner wall. After adding a buffer solution containing water-soluble drugs and shaking, multilameller vesicle will be formed.

(3) Reversed-phase evaporation method Lip-soluble components, such as phospholipid, are

dissolved in organic solvents (such as chloroform), then mixed and emulsified with the buffer containing drugs, and then evaporated under reduced pressure to form liposomes, which are suitable for water-soluble macromolecular active substances with high encapsulation efficiency.

(4) Freeze-drying method Suitable for preparation of labile drug liposomes in water.

(5) Melting method The prepared liposomes are heterogeneous liposomes, which are stable in nature and can be heat sterilized.

4. The encapsulation rate is an important index for evaluating the intrinsic quality of liposomes. Common methods for determining the encapsulation rate include molecular sieve method, ultracentrifugation method, ultrafiltration membrane method and cation exchange resin method.

 Equipments and Materials

1. Equipment Beaker, balance, magnetic stirrer, microscope.

2. Materials Berberine hydrochloride, soybeen phospholipid, cholesterol, ether, disodium hydrogen phosphate, sodium dihydrogen phosphate, distilled water.

 Experimental Procedures

（Ⅰ）Preparation of Liposomes

Berberine Hydrochloride Liposomes

【Formula】

Berberine hydrochloride solution ($1mg \cdot ml^{-1}$)	25ml
Soybeen phospholipid	0.75g
Cholesterol	0.25g
Diethyl ether	35ml

To make 25ml liposomes

【Preparation】

(1) Preparation of phosphate buffered saline (PBS) Weigh 3.7g of disodium hydrogen phosphate ($Na_2HPO_4 \cdot 12H_2O$) and 20g of sodium dihydrogen phosphate ($NaH_2PO_4 \cdot 2H_2O$), add an appropriate amount of distilled water, heat to dissolve, and dilute to 1000ml to obtain $0.067mol \cdot L^{-1}$ phosphate buffer liquid (pH is about 5.7).

(2) Preparation of berberine hydrochloride solution An appropriate amount of berberine hydrochloride was weighed, and $0.067mol \cdot L^{-1}$ phosphate buffer solution was used to prepare a $1mg \cdot ml^{-1}$ solution.

(3) Preparation of berberine hydrochloride liposomes Weigh the prescribed amount of soybeen phospholipid and cholesterol into a 150ml small beaker, add 35ml of ether, stir and dissolve on a magnetic stirrer, add 25ml ($1mg \cdot ml^{-1}$) of berberine hydrochloride solution, continue stirring and emulsify until Ether dilutes into a yellow emulsion, which is the berberine hydrochloride liposomes.

131

Experiment flow chart (Figure 16–1):

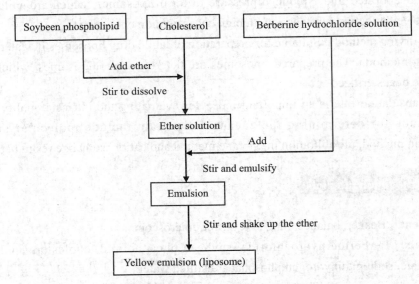

Figure 16–1 Preparation procedure of liposome

【Characters】This product is a uniform yellow emulsion.

【Considerations】

(1) During the injection method experiment, the temperature can be controlled at 50~60°C, and the stirring is always accompanied during the operation. The stirring time after adding the berberine hydrochloride solution must not be less than 2h. Due to the process of liposome formation, the temperature, the drop acceleration and stirring time has an effect on the formation of liposomes.

(2) The ether solution dissolving the phospholipids and cholesterol should be clarified. Otherwise, the impurities should be removed by filtration.

(3) The particle size of liposomes directly affects its distribution in the body. Therefore, it is necessary to ensure that the particle size of liposomes does not change during storage. The following two methods can be used: ① Increasing the zeta potential of the liposomes makes it difficult for the liposome to agglutinate and increase the stability of the liposomes, because the larger the zeta potential, the more the charge on the liposomes surface, and the electrostatic repulsion is also greater, so when preparing liposomes, adding charged lipid components can reduce particle size changes to a minimum. ② The freeze-drying method can improve the physical and chemical stability of liposomes.

(Ⅱ) Determination of Encapsulation Rate of Berberine Hydrochloride Liposomes

1. Preparation of cation exchange resin separation column Weigh about 1.5g of the treated cation-exchange resin, put it in a 5ml syringe barrel with a small amount of glass wool at the bottom, add PBS hydrated cation-exchange resin the cation exchange resin, and drip the PBS naturally to obtain.

2. Investigation of column resolution

(1) Preparation of blank liposomes Weigh 0.9g of soy phospholipid and 0.3g of cholesterol in a small beaker, add 10ml of ether, stir to dissolve, rotate the small beaker to form a film of ether on the wall of the cup, blow with an ear ball, and remove the ether. Take another 30ml of phosphate buffer solution in a small beaker, put it on a magnetic stirrer, and heat it to 55~65°C for later use. Take 20ml of pre-heated phosphate buffer solution into a small beaker containing phospholipid and cholesterol to form a film, then place the small beaker on a magnetic stirrer, keep it at 55~60°C for 10 minutes, and then stir at the same

temperature for 30~60 min (reduced solution volume, added PBS), that's it.

(2) Preparation of mixed solution of berberine hydrochloride and blank liposome $3mg \cdot ml^{-1}$ of berberine hydrochloride solution was accurately measured to take 0.1ml, placed in a small test tube, 0.2ml blank liposome was added, and mixed to obtain.

(3) Preparation of reference solution   Take 0.1ml of mixed solution of berberine hydrochloride and blank liposome into a 10ml volumetric flask, add 6ml of 95% ethanol, shake to dissolve it, add PBS to the mark, and shake to obtain.

(4) Preparation of sample solution   Take 0.1ml of the mixed solution berberine hydrochloride and blank liposomes to the top of the separation column. After the liquid on the top of the column disappears, leave it for 5 minutes, carefully add PBS (note that the ion exchange resin on the top of the column cannot be washed away), and wash remove (about 1.5~2ml PBS), collect the eluate in a 10ml volumetric flask, add 6ml of 95% ethanol and shake to dissolve, add PBS to the scale, shake well, filter, discard the initial filtrate, take the subsequent filtrate was the sample solution.

(5) Preparation of blank solvent   Take 30ml of 95% ethanol, put it into a 50ml measuring flask, add PBS to the mark, and shake it to obtain.

(6) Determination of absorbance   Using the blank solvent as a control, the absorbance of the sample solution and the reference solution was measured at a wavelength of 345nm, and the column resolution was calculated. The resolution is required to be greater than 0.95.

$$\text{Column separation} = \frac{1 - A_{\text{sample}}}{(A_{\text{reference}} \times 2.5)} \tag{16-1}$$

In the formula 16-1, sample A: the absorbance of the sample solution; reference A: the absorbance of the reference solution; 2.5: the dilution factor of the reference solution.

3. Determination of test article   Precision berberine hydrochloride liposomes were taken in two 0.1ml portions, one was placed in a 10ml volumetric flask, and the operation was performed under (2)~(3) under "2.Investigation of column resolution"; the other was placed in a separation column at the top, operate according to (4) under "2.Investigation of column resolution", and measure the absorbance at the wavelength of 345nm, and calculate the encapsulation rate according to the formula 16-2.

$$\text{Encapsulation rate} = \frac{A_{\text{L}}}{A_{\text{r}}} \times 100\% \tag{16-2}$$

In the formula 16-2, A_{L}: the absorbance of the drug after the column separation (in the liposome); A_{r}: the total absorbance of the drug in the test product (in the liposome).

(III) Quality Inspection of Liposomes

1. Particle size and morphology   Observe the particle size and morphology of the liposomes with a microscope. It is a multi-layered capsule or multi-layered sphere, most particle sizes are between 0.7 and 1.2μm.

2. Determination of encapsulation rate   After measuring the total drug amount in liposomes, the liposomes are separated by an appropriate method. The amount of drug encapsulated in the liposomes and the amount of drug unencapsulated in the medium were measured separately, and the encapsulation rate was calculated according to the formula 16-3 and 16-4.

$$\text{Encapsulation rate} = \frac{(\text{Total drug} - \text{Unencapsulated dose in the medium})}{\text{Total drug}} \times 100\% \tag{16-3}$$

$$\text{Encapsulation rate} = \frac{\text{Encapsulated dose in liposomes}}{\text{(Encapsulated dose in liposomes + Unencapsulated dose in the medium)}} \times 100\%$$

(16–4)

3. Leakage rate Depending on the route of administration, the liposomes are dispersedly stored in a certain medium, maintained at a certain temperature, and separated at different times. The amount of drug in the medium is measured, compared with the amount of drug encapsulated before storage, and calculated according to the following formula 16–5 leak age rate.

$$\text{Leakage rate} = \frac{\text{Dose leaking into the medium after storage}}{\text{Encapsulated dose before storage}} \times 100\%$$

(16–5)

4. Residual organic solvents According to the residual solvent determination method in the current edition of the General Principles of the *Chinese Pharmacopoeia*, the determination of organic solvent residues in liposomes should meet the requirements.

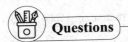 **Questions**

1. What is the purpose of adding cholesterol when preparing liposomes?
2. What are the precautions when adding drugs to the matrix?
3. What is the key to the preparation of liposomes by injection?
4. What are the mechanisms and characteristics of liposomes as carriers of anticancer drugs?

实验十七 微囊的制备

实验目的

1. **掌握** 复凝聚法制备微囊的制备过程。
2. **熟悉** 微囊大小的表征方法。
3. **了解** 影响成囊的主要因素。

实验提要

1. 微囊是利用天然、半合成或合成的高分子材料（通称囊材），将固体或液体药物（通称囊心物）包裹而成直径 1~250μm 的微小胶囊。粒径在 0.1~1μm 的微囊称为亚微囊，粒径在 10~100nm 的微囊称纳米囊。

2. 根据临床需要，可将微囊制成片剂、胶囊剂、注射剂、眼用制剂、鼻腔用制剂、贴剂及喷雾剂等，用微囊制备的制剂均应符合其制剂通则的相关要求。

3. 微囊具有掩盖药物的不良气味与口味，液态药物固态化，减少复方药物的配伍变化，提高难溶性药物的溶解度，或提高药物的生物利用度，或改善药物的稳定性，或降低药物不良反应，或延缓药物释放、提高药物靶向性等优点。

4. 常用的囊材可分为以下 3 类。

（1）天然材料 在体内生物相容和可生物降解，如明胶、白蛋白、壳聚糖、海藻酸盐、阿拉伯胶等。

（2）半合成材料 主要包括乙基纤维素、羧甲纤维素盐、羟丙甲纤维素等。

（3）合成材料 分为在体内可生物降解与不可生物降解两类。可生物降解材料应用较广的有聚乳酸、聚氨基酸、乙交酯 – 丙交酯共聚物等；不可生物降解的材料有聚酰胺、聚乙烯醇、丙烯酸树脂、硅橡胶等。

此外，制备时，可加入适宜的润湿剂、乳化剂、抗氧剂或表面活性剂等。

5. 微囊的制备方法有很多，可归纳为物理化学法、物理机械法和化学法三类。物理化学法，又称相分离法，主要包括凝聚法、液中干燥法、溶剂 – 非溶剂法等。物理机械法主要包括锅包衣法、喷雾干燥法、喷雾冻凝法及流化床包衣法等。化学法包括界面缩聚法和辐射交联法。

凝聚法是最早的微囊化方法之一，主要包括三个步骤：第一步是囊心物、囊材和分散介质三相体系的制备，囊心物分散在囊材溶液中；第二步是囊材的沉积；第三步是囊材的固化。基于微囊化过程中使用的成囊材料的数量不同，凝聚法又可分为单凝聚法和复凝聚法。

单凝聚法：微囊化中只使用一种成囊材料（如明胶、PVA、羧甲基纤维素等），将囊心物分散在囊材中，然后加入凝聚剂，如乙醇、丙酮、二氧六环、异丙醇和丙醇等亲水性非电解质，或硫酸钠、硫酸铵等强亲水性电解质，或者通过改变温度等，由于凝聚剂与囊材水合膜的水结合，致使囊材的溶解度降低而凝聚形成微囊。

复凝聚法：利用两种具有相反电荷的亲水性高分子材料作为囊材，当两种相反电荷的胶体溶液混合时，对体系中和而产生凝聚，经典的复合囊材是明胶－阿拉伯胶体系。由于静电作用的参与，对体系 pH 的控制非常重要。如阿拉伯胶带负电荷，明胶在等电点（pH 4.5）以上带负电荷而在等电点以下带正电荷，因此，在等电点以下，带正电荷的明胶可与带负电荷的阿拉伯胶凝聚，包囊药物而成微囊。

　　囊心物的溶解度、囊材的溶解度和浓度、成囊温度、搅拌速度及 pH 等因素对成囊过程和成品质量均有重要影响，制备时应严格把握成囊条件。微囊化方法的选择主要考虑囊心物的性质，囊材的选择要尽可能满足囊心物性质的要求。

实验器材

1. 仪器　恒温磁力搅拌器、水浴锅、研钵、温度计、显微镜、烧杯、组织捣碎机、pH 计、制冰机、电子天平、量筒、移液管等。

2. 试药　薄荷油、明胶、阿拉伯胶、甲醛、醋酸、氢氧化钠、液状石蜡等。

实验操作步骤

复凝聚法制备薄荷油微囊

【处方】

薄荷油	2ml
阿拉伯胶	5g
明胶	5g
10% 醋酸溶液	适量
37% 甲醛溶液	2.5ml
10% 氢氧化钠溶液	适量
蒸馏水	适量

【制法】微囊的制备工艺流程图如图 17-1 所示。

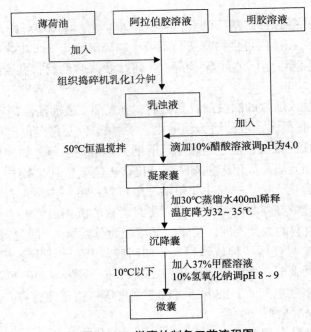

图 17-1　微囊的制备工艺流程图

（1）明胶溶液的配制　取明胶 5g，先加适量水浸泡溶胀至溶解，再于 60℃水浴中至完全溶解，加水至 100ml，搅匀，备用。

（2）阿拉伯胶溶液的配制　取蒸馏水 80ml 至小烧杯中，将 5g 阿拉伯胶粉末撒于液面，待粉末润湿下沉后，加热至 80℃左右，轻轻搅拌使溶解，加蒸馏水至 100ml，搅匀，备用。

（3）薄荷油乳的制备　取薄荷油 2ml 与 5% 阿拉伯胶溶液 100ml 至组织捣碎机中，乳化 1 分钟即得到乳浊液。取乳浊液一滴，至载玻片上镜检，绘制乳剂形态图。

（4）微囊的制备　将乳浊液转移至 1000ml 烧杯中，加 100ml 明胶溶液，于 50℃水浴上恒温搅拌；滴加 10% 醋酸溶液调节 pH 为 4.0，使明胶凝聚；加入 400ml 30℃ 的蒸馏水稀释凝聚囊，待体系温度降为 32~35℃时，将微囊液置于冰浴搅拌降温至 10℃；加入 37% 甲醛溶液 2.5ml，搅拌 15 分钟；用 10% 氢氧化钠溶液调 pH 至 8.0~9.0，继续搅拌 20 分钟，观察至微囊析出为止；静置，待微囊沉降，过滤干燥即得。

【质量检查】微囊形态、大小表征的质量检查如下。

（1）形态　取少量微囊混悬液，置于载玻片上，显微镜上观察微囊形态图。

（2）粒径大小及分布　采用光学显微镜法测量粒径大小及分布。至少需要测量 500 个微囊粒子，然后通过计算机软件计算其平均粒径。粒径分布数据，常用各粒径范围内的粒子数或百分率表示。如需作图，则将所测得的粒径分布数据，以粒径为横坐标，以频率（每一粒径范围的粒子个数除以粒子总数所得的百分率）为纵坐标，即得粒径分布直方图。

【性状】显微镜下观察，微囊形状较为圆整。

【注意事项】

（1）纯化水的使用　为避免粒子对凝聚的干扰，实验中要使用纯化水。

（2）成囊时的搅拌速度　成囊时搅拌的速度与囊粒大小关系密切，搅拌快而囊粒小，搅拌慢而囊粒大。但用明胶包裹不宜快速搅拌，否则会产生大量气泡，影响得率，搅拌速度应以产生气泡最少为度。必要时还可加几滴戊醇或辛醇作为消泡剂。

（3）固化交联和搅拌　固化交联时为避免微囊间的粘连，应持续搅拌。

（4）加入 400ml 蒸馏水　其目的主要是稀释凝聚囊，避免相互干扰，使所得微囊具有完整的外形。

思考题

1. 制备微囊的方法有哪些？
2. 复凝聚法制备微囊中影响微囊成型的主要因素有哪些？

题库

Experiment 17　Preparation of Microcapsules

Purposes

1. To master the process for preparation of microcapsules by complex coacervation.
2. To be familiar with the method for determining the size of microcapsules by optical microscopy.
3. To understand the factors that affect the encapsulation efficiency.

Introduction

1. Microcapsules are extra fine capsules produced by coating solid or liquid drug materials with a thin layer of excipients. Microcapsules consist of two components, namely core material and coating of shell material. Core material contains an active ingredient while inert coating or shell material covers or protects the core material. Usually their size ranges from 1μm to 250μm, while those with size ranging from 0.1μm to 1μm are called sub-microcapsules, and from 10nm to 100nm called nanocapsules.

2. Microcapsules can be used as drug carriers. Preparations of microcapsules should conform to the general requirements for the corresponding preparations, such as tablets, capsules, injections, ophthalmic preparations, nasal preparations, patches, and aerosols, etc.

3. Transformation of drugs into microcapsules can mask their unpleasant smell and taste, enhance stability, prevent the drug from deactivation in stomach or lessen their irritancy to stomach, and facilitate transportation. Microencapsulation can also solidify liquid drugs, improve compatibility of drugs or excipients in compound preparations and helps the preparations achieve sustained, controlled and delayed release, for some of them, targeting release characteristics.

4. Usually coating of shell material in common use is generally classified into three types.

(1) Natural materials: Bioconsistent and biodegradable natural materials include gelatin, albumin, alginate, chitosan, acacia, etc.

(2) Semisynthesized materials: They include ethylcellulose, carboxymethyl-cellulosesalt, and hydroxypropylmethyl cellulose, etc.

(3) Synthesized materials: They are divided into two types (biodegradable and nonbiodegradable materials). The most widely used biodegradable materials include poly-lacticacid, poly-amino acid, and poly-lactide-glycolide, etc. Non-biodegradable materials include polyamide, polyvinyl alcohol, eudragin, and silicon rubber, etc.

In addition, wetting agents, emulsifiers, antioxidants or surfactants can be added for preparing microcapsules.

5. Microencapsulation techmology can be categorized into three types. This includes physico-chemical methods, physical mechanical methods and chemical methods. Physico-chemical methods, also

known as phase separation methods, include coacervation phase separation, in-liquid drying and solvent-non-solvent, etc. Physical-mechanical methods include pan coating, spray drying, spray congealing and air suspension coating, etc. Chemical methods include interfacial polymerization and radiation crosslinking.

The coacervation phase separation is one of the earliest microencapsulation techniques. The process of coacervation can be divided into three basic steps. The first step involves the information of three immiscible phases (liquid manufacturing vehicle, core material and coating material). The core material is dispersed in a solution of the cating polymer. The second step includes deposition of liquid polymers upon the core material. Finally, the prepared microcapsules are stabilized by cross-linking, desolvation or thermal treatment. Cross-linking is the formation of chemical links between molecular chains to form a three-dimensional network of connected molecules. Coacervation can be achieved by simple or complex coacervation, depending on the number of polymers that are involved in the formation of microparticles.

Simple coacervation: This process involves only one polyer (e.g., gelatin, polyvinyl alcohol, carboxymethyl cellulose) as coating material, and phase separation can be induced by conditions that result in desolvation (or dehydration) of the polymer phase. These conditions include addition of a water-miscible co-solvent, such as ethanol, acetone, dioxane, isopropanol, or propanol, or addition of inorganic salts, such as sodium sulfate, or through temperature change.

Complex coacervation: This process involves two hydrophilic polymers of opposite charges. Neutralization of the overall positively charged polymers by the negatively charged polyer is used to bring about separation of the polymer-rich phase. The best-known example is the gelatin-acacia system. Since electrostatic interactions are involved, the pH of the medium is very important. For example, in the gelatin-acacia system, pH should be below the isoelectric point (pH 4.5) of gelatin so that the gelatin can maintain positively charged, which interact with the oppositely charged acacia. Once embryonic coacervates form around the dispersed oil or solid phases, these polymer complexes can be stabilized by cross-linking using formaldehyde.

There are many factors affecting the encapsulation efficiency. This includes, solubility of polymer in solvent, concentration of polymer, solubility of core material in the continuous phase, temperature, pH and stirring speed, etc. In selection of the microencapsulation methods for a given drug, it is important to understand the physicochemical properties of the drug and select a method and polymeric materials that best match the properties.

 Equipments and Materials

1. Equipments Constant temperature magnetic stirrer, water bath pot, mortar, thermometer, microscopy, beaker, homogenizer, pH meter, ice maker, electronic balance, cylinder, pipette, etc.

2. Materials Peppermint oil, gelatin, acacia, formaldehyde, acetic acid, sodium hydroxide, liquid paraffin, etc.

 Experimental Procedures

Preparation of Microcapsules of Peppermint Oil by the Complex Coacervation
【Formula】
Peppermint oil   2ml

Acacia	5g
Gelatin	5g
Acetic acid solution (10%)	q.s.
Formaldehyde solution (37%)	2.5ml
Sodium hydroxide solution (10%)	q.s.
Distilled water	q.s.

【 Preparation 】

(1) Preparation of gelatin solution: Take 5g of gelatin, and dissolve it in a small amount of purified water by heating in a 60℃ water bath. Add more water to the resultant solution to make up a final volume of 100ml. Mix the solution until it is uniform for use.

(2) Preparation of acacia solution: 5g of acacia powder is suspended in 80ml of distilled water. The resultant mixture is heated to about 80℃ under gently stirring until the acacia is completely dissolved. Add water to make up a final volume of 100ml and mix well.

(3) Peppermint oil emulsion: 2ml of peppermint is emulsified with 100ml of a 5% acacia solution by homogenizer for 1 min. Observe the morphology of the emulsion under an optical microscope. Draw a picture to illustrate the morphology.

(4) Microencapsulation: Peppermint oil emulsion is transferred into a 1000ml beaker, and 100ml of 5% gelatin solution is added into the emulsion. Mix the resultant mixture by stirring gently while kept in a 50℃ water bath. Adjust the pH of the mixture to pH 4.0 using 10% acetic acid solution, followed by adding 400ml of distilled water (30℃). Remove the mixture from the water bath and let it cooled at room temperature under constant stirring until the temperature is in the range 32~35℃. The temperature of the mixture is further lower to below 10℃ with an ice bath. Add 2.5ml of 37% formaldehyde solution dropwise to the mixture and keep continuously stirring for 15 min. The pH of the system is adjusted to 8.0~9.0 using a 10% sodium hydroxide solution, followed by continuous stirring for 20 min. Stop stirring to allow the microcapsules to settle undisturbed. The aqueous phase is removed by decanting and the microcapsules are collected by filtration. The collected microcapsules are rewashed and dried under vacuum.

Experiment flow chart (Figure 17-1):

【 Quality Inspection 】 Quality inspection of morphology, size and distribution of microcapsules.

(1) Morphology observation   The moist microcapsules are suspended in the water and observed by optical microscopy.

(2) Size and distribution   The average value of particle size and the data or graphs of its distribution can be determined using an optical microscope. A minimum of 500 microcapsules must be measured, and computer software can be used to calculate the arithmetic average diameter.If needed, particle size distribution can be graphically described by plotting the particle size interval as abscissa against the frequency (the percentage of particle numbers in different size ranges in the total number of the particles) as the ordinate to produce a histogram.

【 Characters 】 The shape of the microcapsule is relatively complete if it was observed by microscope.

【 Considerations 】

(1) Purified water   To avoid the interference with coacervation by ions, purified water should be used.

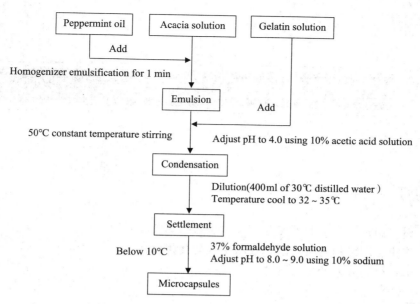

Figure 17-1   Preparation procedure of microcapsule

(2) Agitation speed   During the microencapsulation, the mixture should be stirred slowly to avoid foam formation. The optimum rate of stirring is based on the minimum bubbling formation. If needed, a small amount (severa drops) of pentanol or octanol can be added as the deforming agent.

(3) Stirring during cross-linking   Do not stop stirring before cross-linking is completed to prevent microcapsules from adhering to each other.

(4) Purpose of adding 400ml of distilled water   It is dilute the coagulated microcapsules and to improve their shape.

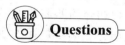 **Questions**

1. What are the preparation metheds of microcapsules?

2. What are the key factors influencing the formation of microcapsules when the complex coacervation method is used?

实验十八 固体制剂的溶出度测定

PPT

实验目的

1. **掌握** 固体制剂溶出度的测定原理、方法与数据处理。
2. **熟悉** 溶出度测定的意义,溶出度测定仪的使用方法。
3. **了解** 溶出仪的基本构造与性能。

实验提要

1. 溶出度系指活性药物从片剂、胶囊剂或颗粒剂等普通制剂在规定条件下溶出的速率和程度,在缓释制剂、控释制剂、肠溶制剂及透皮贴剂等制剂中也称释放度。溶出度是评价药物口服固体制剂质量的重要指标,是一种模拟口服固体制剂在胃肠道中崩解和溶出的体外简易实验方法。

2. 溶出度的测定原理为 Noyes—Whitney 方程:

$$dc/dt = ks(C_s - C_t)$$

式中,dc/dt 为溶出速度;k 为溶出速度常数;s 为固体药物表面积;C_s 为药物的饱和溶液浓度;C_t 为 t 时溶液的药物浓度。实验中,溶出介质的量必须远远超过使药物饱和的介质所需要的量。通常以固体制剂中主药溶出一定量所需时间或规定时间内主药溶出百分数作为制剂质量评价指标。

3. 《中国药典》2020 年版四部通则 0931 规定的"溶出度与释放测定法"有第一法(转篮法)、第二法(桨法)、第三法(小杯法)、第四法(桨碟法)和第五法(转筒法)。常用的溶出介质有人工胃液、人工肠液、蒸馏水,有时还需要加入适量的表面活性剂等。操作容器为 1000ml 圆底烧杯,第三法采用 250ml 圆底烧杯。第一法与第二法规定转速为每分钟 50~200 转,第三法规定转速为每分钟 25~200 转,第四法规定溶出杯中放入用于放置贴片的不锈钢网碟,第五法规定搅拌桨另用不锈钢转筒装置代替。

4. 在固体制剂溶出度研究中,常每隔一定时间取样一次,测定一系列时间药物溶出百分数,对实验数据进行数学模型拟合,求算特征溶出度参数,用以描述药物制剂在体外溶出或释放的规律。常用数学模型有单指数模型、Higuchi 方程、Weibull 概率模型,以及用于溶出曲线相似性比较的变异因子与相似因子等。

实验器材

1. **仪器** 溶出度测定仪(第一法)、分析天平、量筒、容量瓶、水浴锅、注射器、微孔滤膜、紫外–可见分光光度计等。

2. **试药** 人工胃液、牛黄解毒片、蒸馏水等。

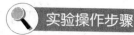 **实验操作步骤**

（一）牛黄解毒片中黄芩苷溶出度的测定

1. E 值的测定　取牛黄解毒片 10 片，精密称定，计算出平均片重（$\overline{W}$），将称定的药片研细，再精密称取相当于 $\overline{W}$ 的量，置 1000ml 容量瓶中，加入人工胃液至刻度，混匀，放于 37℃±0.5℃ 水浴中，不时振摇，浸渍 24 小时，取样，滤过，用紫外 – 可见分光光度计于 276nm 处测定吸收度 E 值。

2. 样品 E_i 值的测定　取温度为 37℃±0.5℃ 的人工胃液 1000ml，倒入圆底烧杯中，调节转篮转速为每分钟 100 转，将精密称重的药片 1 片（W_1）放在转篮内，以人工胃液接触药片开始计时，每隔 10 分钟取样一次（取样位置固定在转篮正中，距杯壁不小于 1cm 处），每次取样 10ml，并立即补充新鲜人工胃液 10ml 于圆底烧杯中。取出的样品液滤过后用紫外 – 可见分光光度计于 276nm 处测定吸收度 E_i 值。

（二）实验数据处理

1. 测得结果记录　牛黄解毒片实验结果记入表 18-1 中，并计算百分溶出量和残留待溶量。

表 18-1　牛黄解毒片中黄芩苷溶出度测定数据及计算结果

取样时间 /min	空白	10	20	30	40	50	60	70	80	90	100
E_i											
百分溶出量 /%											
残留待溶量 /%											

［注］百分溶出量（%）$=\dfrac{\overline{W}E_i}{W_iE}\times100\%$；残留待溶量（%）=1– 百分溶出量。

2. 溶出曲线　以百分溶出量为纵坐标，溶出时间为横坐标得到溶出曲线。

3. 用 Weibull 概率模型拟合，求溶出参数 $T_{0.5}$、T_d 及 m　Weibull 分布函数的数学表达式如式（18-1）：

$$F(t) = 1 - e^{-\frac{(t-\alpha)^m}{\beta}} \tag{18-1}$$

对式（18-1）进行两次取对数后，得到式（18-2）：

$$\ln\ln\frac{1}{1-F(t)} = m\ln(t-\alpha) - \ln\beta \tag{18-2}$$

固体剂型溶出度试验中，通常 $\alpha=0$，因此式（18-2）可简化为式（18-3）：

$$\ln\ln\frac{1}{1-F(t)} = m\ln t - \ln\beta \tag{18-3}$$

用于溶出度试验时，式中，t 为取样时间；$F(t)$ 为百分溶出量；m 为形状参数；β 为尺度参数。可见 $\ln\ln\dfrac{1}{1-F(t)}$ 与 $\ln t$ 之间存在线性关系，拟合后可求得 m 以及 $T_{0.5}$（溶出 50% 所需时间）、T_d（溶出 63.2% 所需时间）。将表 18-1 的数据依次转换，填于表 18-2。

表 18-2　Weibull 概率数据表

取样时间 /min t	百分溶出量 /min $F(t)$	$\ln t$	$\dfrac{1}{1-F(t)}$	$\ln\dfrac{1}{1-F(t)}$	$\ln\ln\dfrac{1}{1-F(t)}$
10					
20					
30					
40					
50					
60					
70					
80					
90					
100					

　　优选 $F(t)$ 在 30%~70% 范围的数据，以 $\ln\ln\dfrac{1}{1-F(t)}$ 对 $\ln t$ 进行拟合，得拟合方程。拟合方程的斜率为 m；令拟合方程中 $F(t)=50\%$，可求得 $T_{0.5}$；令拟合方程中 $F(t)=63.2\%$，可求得 T_d。

思考题

1. 哪些药物应进行溶出度测定？
2. 影响溶出度测定结果的因素主要有哪些？

Experiment 18 — Dissolution Test of Solid Preparations

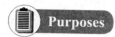 **Purposes**

1. To master the determination principle, method and data handling of dissolution of solid preparation.

2. To be familiar with the significance of the dissolution test and the usage of dissolution test analyzer.

3. To understand the basic structure and performance of dissolution test analyzer.

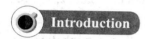 **Introduction**

1. Dissolution refers to the dissolution rate and degree of active pharmaceutical ingredients from dosage forms such as tablets, capsules or granules under the specified conditions, which is also known as release in sustained-release preparation, controlled-release preparation, enteric-coated preparation or transdermal patches. Dissolution is an important index to evaluate the quality of oral solid preparation. It is simple in vitro test to simulate the disintegration and dissolution of oral solid preparation in the gastrointestinal tract.

2. The determination principle of dissolution is the Noyes-Whitney equation:

$$dc/dt = ks(C_s - C_t)$$

Where, dc/dt is dissolution rate, k is dissolution rate constant, s is surface area of solid preparations, C_s is saturated concentration of the drug, C_t is drug concentration at t. In the test, the volume of dissolution medium must far exceed the volume needed to saturate the drug. The time required to dissolute certain amounts of the active pharmaceutical ingredients from solid preparations or dissolution rate of the active pharmaceutical ingredients within a given time is usually used as the evaluation index of the preparation quality.

3. The General rule 0931 "Dissolution and Release Test" of *Chinese Pharmacopoeia* 2020 edition (Vol. IV) includes Method 1 (Basket method), Method 2 (Paddle method), Method 3 (Small cup method), Method 4 (Paddle over disk method) and Method 5 (Rotating-cylinder method). The commonly used dissolution media includes artificial gastric juice, artificial intestinal juice, distilled water, and sometimes proper quantity of surfactants are also needed. The operating vessel is a 1000ml beaker. A 250ml beaker is required in Method 3. Agitation rates between 50 and 200 rpm are required in Method 1 and Method 2, and between 25 and 200 rpm are required in Method 3. A stainless steel disk is required to be placed in the vessel for placing the patch in Method 4. The paddle is replaced by a stainless steel rotating-cylinder in Method 5.

4. In the study of dissolution for solid preparation, samples are usually taken at a regular time interval to determine the amount dissolved from preparations over a period of time, the experimental data

145

are fitted by mathematical model, and the characteristic dissolution parameters are calculated to describe the rule of dissolution or release of preparations *in vitro*. Conventional mathematical models include single index model, Higuchi equation, Weibull probability model, and variation factors and similarity factors for similarity comparison of dissolution curve.

 Equipments and Materials

1. Equipments Dissolution test analyzer (Method 1), analytical balance, cylinder, volumetric flask, water bath, syringe, microporous membrane, ultraviolet spectrophotometer, etc.

2. Materials Artificial gastric juice, Niuhuang Jiedu Tablets, distilled water, etc.

 Experimental Procedures

(I) Determination of the Dissolution of Baicalin in Niuhuang Jiedu Tablets

1. Determination of base E Weigh accurately 10 pieces of Niuhuang Jiedu Tablets and calculate the average weight of one tablet ($\overline{W}$), grind into powder, weigh accurately $\overline{W}$ to a 1000ml volumetric flask, add artificial gastric juice to volume and mix well. In a water bath at 37℃±0.5℃ for 24 hours, sample and filter, measure the absorbance of the filtrate (the value of base E) at 276nm by UV spectrophotometer.

2. Determination of sample E_i Place 1000ml of artificial gastric juice (37℃±0.5℃) in the vessel (a beaker), adjust the rotating speed of the basket to 100 rpm, place one tablet (W_1) into the basket. Start the counting of time when artificial gastric juice contact table, withdraw 10ml of solution every 10 minutes, filter, and replace the samples withdrawn with equal volumes of fresh artificial gastric juice (Withdraw an aliquot of solution from a zone midway of the rotating basket, not less than 1cm apart from the wall of vessel). Measure the absorbance of the filtrate (the value of sample E_i) at 276nm by UV spectrophotometer.

(II) Experimental Data Handling

1. Record the measurement results Record experimental results of Niuhuang Jiedu Tablets in the Table18-1, and calculate the amount of baicalin dissolved from tablet (Percentage of accumulated dissolution) and the residual amount of baicalin undissolved from table (Percentage of undissolution).

Table 18-1　Determination data and results of baicalin dissolution in Niuhuang Jiedu Tablets

Sampling time/min	Blank	10	20	30	40	50	60	70	80	90	100
E_i											
Percentage of accumulated dissolution/%											
Percentage of undissolution /%											

[Note] Percentage of accumulated dissolution (%) = $\dfrac{\overline{W}E_i}{W_iE} \times 100\%$, Percentage of undissolution (%) = 1−Percentage of accumulated dissolution.

2. Dissolution curve The dissolution curve is obtained by taking the percentage of accumulated dissolution as ordinate and the dissolution time as abscissa.

3. Obtain dissolution parameters $T_{0.5}$、T_d and m by fitting the Weibull probability model The mathematical expression of the Weibull distribution function is shown in equation (18–1).

$$F(t) = 1 - e^{-\frac{(t-\alpha)^m}{\beta}}$$
(18–1)

Take the logarithm of equation (18–1) twice, obtain equation (18–2).

$$\ln \ln \frac{1}{1-F(t)} = m \ln(t-\alpha) - \ln \beta$$
(18–2)

In the dissolution test of solid preparations, usually, $\alpha=0$, so equation (18–2) can be simplified to equation (18–3).

$$\ln \ln \frac{1}{1-F(t)} = m \ln t - \ln \beta$$
(18–3)

Where, t is sampling time, $F(t)$ is percentage of accumulated dissolution, m is the shape parameter, and β is the scale parameter. There is a linear relationship between $\ln \ln \frac{1}{1-F(t)}$ and $\ln t$, and m, $T_{0.5}$ (time to dissolve 50%) and T_d (time to dissolve 63.2%) can be obtained by fitting. Convert the data in the Table 18–1 and fill them in Table 18–2.

Table 18–2   Weibull probability data table

Sampling time/min t	Percentage of accumulated dissolution/% $F(t)$	$\ln t$	$\frac{1}{1-F(t)}$	$\ln \frac{1}{1-F(t)}$	$\ln \ln \frac{1}{1-F(t)}$
10					
20					
30					
40					
50					
60					
70					
80					
90					
100					

Prioritize $F(t)$ in the range of 30%~70%, obtain the fitting equation by fitting $\ln t$ with $\ln \ln \frac{1}{1-F(t)}$. The slope of the fitting equation is m. Obtain $T_{0.5}$ when $F(t)$=50% and T_d when $F(t)$=63.2%.

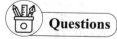 **Questions**

1. Which kinds of drugs should be tested for dissolution?
2. What are the main factors that affect the results of dissolution determination?

实验十九　中药缓释制剂释放度的测定

实验目的

1. **掌握**　缓释制剂的释放原理及中药缓释制剂释放度的测定方法。
2. **熟悉**　中药缓释制剂的质量控制指标。

实验提要

1. 缓释制剂系指口服药物在规定溶剂中，按要求缓慢地非恒速释放。缓释制剂的优点是可以减少给药次数，并使血药浓度保持在比较平稳持久。中药缓释制剂是中药现代化研究的一项重要内容。缓释制剂按剂型分主要有片剂、颗粒剂、微丸、混悬剂、胶囊剂、栓剂等。按照制备技术可以分为整体骨架技术、分数剂量延迟技术和骨架型多层压片技术等。

2. 释放度系指口服药物从缓释制剂、控释制剂、肠溶制剂及透皮贴剂等在规定溶剂中释放的速度和程度。它是评价药物制剂质量的一个内在指标，是一种模拟口服固体制剂在胃肠道中的崩解和溶出的体外试验法。

3. 缓释制剂释药的原理主要基于控制溶出、扩散、溶蚀或扩散与溶出兼备以及渗透压交换等机制。缓释制剂一般应进行释放度检查，测定方法与要求可参照 2020 年版《中国药典》（四部）0931 项下有关规定。常采用转篮法、桨法等。

对于成熟产品，其质量控制主要反映在释放度的测定。中药缓释制剂应选用至少一个指标成分进行释放度的测定。

实验器材

1. **仪器**　乳钵、分析天平、溶出仪、注射器、紫外 – 可见分光光度计、试管、容量瓶、微孔滤膜器（孔径 0.45μm）、移液管。
2. **试药**　正清风痛宁缓释片、纯净水、盐酸青藤碱对照品。

实验操作步骤

（一）释放度检查

取正清风痛宁缓释片按照桨法进行释放度测定，取 900ml 水为介质，在 37.0℃±0.5℃、每分钟 100 转条件下，在预定的时间分别取溶液 5ml 滤过，并即时在操作容器中补充溶剂 5ml。采用紫外 – 可见分光光度法，在 265nm 波长处测定吸收度。另精密称取盐酸青藤碱对照品并配制成浓度为 40μg/ml 的溶液。同法测定吸收度，按标准对照法计算，即得。

实验流程图如图 19-1 所示。

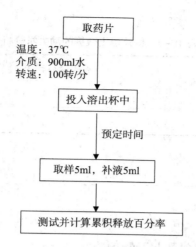

图 19-1　中药缓释制剂释放度测定实验流程图

（二）实验结果与数据处理

1. 释放度及释放曲线　计算各取样时间的药物释放量，并按标示量估算各取样时间的累积释放百分率。以累积释放百分率对时间作图，得释放曲线（表 19-1）。

药物累积释放百分率公式：

$$F = \frac{C_t \times V \times A_t}{M} \times 100\%$$

式中，F 为累积释放百分率；C_t 是 t 时间测试样品浓度；V 是溶出介质总体积；A_t 是 t 时间测试样品稀释倍数；M 是投入药物量。

表 19-1　药物累计释放百分率结果

时间 t/h	累计释放百分率 /%
1	
2	
4	
6	
8	
12	

2. 释药机制　进行以下三种释放数学模型拟合。

零级释放模型：$F = K_0 t$

式中，F 为累计释放百分率；t 为时间；K_0 为零级释放速率常数。

一级释放模型：$\ln(1-F) = K_1 t$

式中，F 为累计释放百分率；t 为时间；K_1 为一级释放速率常数。

Higuchi 模型：$F = K_H t^{1/2}$

式中，F 为累计释放百分率；t 为时间；K_H 为 Higuchi 溶出常数。

分别按上述数学模型方程，对正清风痛宁缓释片的溶出数据进行拟合，结果见表 19-2。

具体计算方法为：将零级释放模型和一级释放模型以横坐标为时间 t，纵坐标分别为累积释放量百分率 F 和 $\ln(1-F)$ 进行直线拟合作图。Higuchi 模型中以横坐标时间 $t_{1/2}$，纵坐标为累计

释放百分率 F，进行直线拟合作图。记录上述三条直线方程的相关系数 R^2。相关系数越接近 1，说明其释放曲线越符合该动力学模型。

表 19-2　体外溶出数据的动力学分析

正清风痛宁缓释片	零级释放模型	一级释放模型	Higuchi 模型
	R^2	R^2	R^2

思考题

1. 缓释制剂的设计原理有哪些？
2. 缓释制剂释放度测定的操作要点主要有哪些？
3. 缓释制剂进行体外释放度检查有何意义？

Experiment 19　*In Vitro* Release Studies of Chinese Medicine Sustained-release Preparation

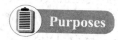

Purposes

1. To master the drug-releasing mechanisms of sustained-release preparation and the procedure of drug release test of Chinese medicine sustained-release preparation.

2. To be familiar with the quality control index of Chinese medicine sustained-release preparation.

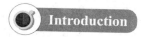

Introduction

1. The sustained-release preparation is preparation which release drug substances in a gradual, non-constant rate way in a specified release medium. The advantage of sustained-release preparation is reducing dosing frequency and controlling the level of drug in blood in a small range for a long time. Chinese medicine sustained-release preparation is one of the most important substances for the modernization of Chinese medicine sustained-release preparation. According to the dosage forms the sustained-release preparation can be divided into tablets, granules, pellets, suspensions, capsules, suppositories and so on. It can also classified into the whole matrix technique, fractional dose delay release technique and matrix multi-layer tablet technique.

2. Drug dissolution is the rate and degree of dissolution of sustained-release preparation, controlled-release preparation, enteric preparation and transdermal patch at specified medium. Drug dissolution is used to be one measure of the quality of preparations as an inner index. It is an *in vitro* test method to simulate the disintegration and dissolution of oral solid preparation in gastrointestinal tract.

3. Drug-releasing mechanisms of sustained-release preparation are based mainly on controlling the mechanisms of dissolution, diffusion, corrosion, or both diffusion and dissolution, as well as osmotic pressure exchange and so on. In general condition, the drug release test should be conducted. The sustained-release preparation should comply with the related requirements for the dissolution and drug-release test (0931) in *China Pharmacopoeia*. The drug-releasing test can be determined by different types of apparatus (Basket apparatus, Paddle apparatus).

For mature products, its quality control was based on drug-releasing test. At least one index composition in the Chinese medicine sustained-release preparation should be selected for drug-release test.

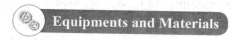

Equipments and Materials

1. Equipments　Pestle, analytical balance, dissolution tester, syringe, ultraviolet spectrophotometer, test tube, volumetric flask, microporous filter membrane filter (0.45μm), pipette.

2. Materials Zhengqingfengtongning sustained-release tablet, water, sinomenine hydrochloride reference substance.

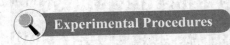

(I) The Release Rate Test

The release rate is determined with the apparatus of dissolution determination paddle method. 900ml distilled water is used as the medium, the rotating rate is 100rpm at 37°C ± 0.5°C. At predetermined time intervals, withdraw a sample of 5ml of the solution, filler through membrane filter, and supply 5ml of water immediately to maintain the volume constant. Measure the absorbance of resulting solutions at 265nm using a UV spectrophotometer. Furthermore, sinomenine hydrochloride reference substance is weighted and prepared in to volumetric flask of 40μg/ml. Measure the absorbance of resulting solutions at 265nm using a UV spectrophotometer. The percentage of cumulative drug release is quantitatively determined by calculating absorbance.

Experiment flow chart (Figure 19–1):

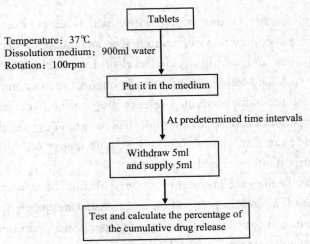

Figure 19–1 Experimental procedure for determination of the *in vitro* release rate of Chinese medicine sustained-release preparations

(Ⅱ) The Experimental Results and Data Processing

1. *In vitro* release rate and the releasing curve Calculate the drug release amount at each sampling time, and estimate the percentage of cumulative drug release of each sampling time (Table 19–1). The release curse can be obtained by plotting the percentage of cumulative drug release verse time.

The percentage of cumulative drug release formula:

$$F = \frac{C_t \times V \times A_t}{M} \times 100\%$$

Where, F stands for the percentage of cumulative drug release, C_t is the test sample concentration at t h, V is the volume of dissolution medium, A_t is the sample dilution multiple at t h, M is the total amount of the drug.

Table 19–1   The data of the percentage of cumulative release

Time/h	Percentage of cumulative release/%
1	
2	
4	
6	
8	
12	

2. Mecanism of drug release   The release data can be generally fitted to the following three math models.

Zero-order equation: $F = K_0 t$

Where F stands for the percentage of cumulative drug release, t is time, K_0 is the release rate constant.

First-order equation: $\ln(1-F) = K_1 t$

Where F stands for the percentage of cumulative drug release, t is time, K_1 is the release rate constant.

Higuchi's equation: $F = K_H t_{1/2}$

Where F stands for the percentage of cumulative drug release, t is time, K_H is the Higuchi release rate constant.

The above math model equation s are used to fit the data of Zheng Qing Feng Tong Ning sustained-release tablet. The results are listed in the Table 19–2.

The calculation methods are as follows: In Excel, the Zero-order equation and the First-order equation curve is fitted by t as X-axis, and F and $\ln(1-F)$ as Y-axis, respectively; The Higuchi's equation curve is fitted by $t_{1/2}$ as X-axis and F as Y-axis. Record the correlation coefficient (R^2) of the above three linear equations. The closer that this value is to 1, the release curve is more consistent with the kinetic model.

Table 19–2   Kinetic analysis of the in vitro release data

Zhengqingfengtongning sustained-release tablets	Zero order	First order	Higuchi
	R^2	R^2	R^2

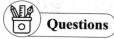 **Questions**

1. What are the design principles of sustained-release preparations?

2. What are the drug release determination of operating points of sustained-release preparations?

3. What is the importance of the test of the drug release determination of sustained-release preparations?

实验二十　药剂的稳定性恒温加速试验

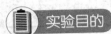 **实验目的**

1. **掌握**　恒温加速实验法预测银黄胶囊有效期的方法。
2. **熟悉**　制剂稳定性考核的项目和方法。
3. **了解**　影响制剂稳定性的因素与稳定化方法。

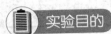 **实验提要**

1. 药剂的稳定性是指药剂从制备、贮运到临床应用，其化学、物理及生物学特性发生变化的程度。稳定性试验是为了考察原料药或药物制剂在处方因素（pH、离子强度、辅料等）和外界因素（温度、湿度、光线等）的影响下随时间变化的规律，为药品的生产、包装、贮运条件提供科学依据，同时通过试验确定药品的有效期。对保障药品临床应用的安全和有效有非常重要的意义。

2. 稳定性试验方法归纳起来有三种，有比较试验法、留样观察法和加速试验法等。比较试验法一般常用于制剂处方组成和制剂工艺设计，而对制剂成品有效期的预测多采用留样观察法和加速试验法。

3. 稳定性试验一般应选择在一定条件（温度、光照、湿度）下制剂中不稳定的活性成分或指标作为考核指标。测定方法应灵敏、准确，能反映加速试验过程中指标成分的浓度（含量）变化，反映制剂的稳定性。

4. 应用化学动力学原理对制剂的稳定性进行加速试验，可加快进度，缩短时间。具体方法有经典恒温法、简便法、经验法和台阶型变温法等。

5. 经典恒温加速试验的理论依据是阿伦尼乌斯（Arrhenius）指数定律。根据化学动力学原理，将样品放入各个不同温度的恒温器中，定时取样测定浓度，得出各温度下不同时间药物的浓度，通过回归法，可推算出室温下样品分解一定程度所需时间。此法可用于制剂处方筛选、工艺改进、有效期预测等，但分析计算量较大。具体实验步骤如下：①确定温度点进行加速试验；②确定反应级数；③求各试验温度的 K 值；④以 $\lg K$ 对 $1/T$ 作图或作线性回归；⑤求算室温（25℃）时的 K 值；⑥求室温时的有效期 $t_{0.9}$ 和半衰期 $t_{1/2}$。

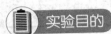 **实验器材**

1. **仪器**　高效液相色谱仪、分析天平、超声提取器、容量瓶、移液管、三角瓶、恒温干燥箱、干燥器。
2. **试药**　银黄胶囊、绿原酸对照品、乙腈（色谱级）、甲醇、磷酸、超纯水。

实验操作步骤

银黄胶囊的稳定性恒温加速试验

【实验操作】

（1）样品处理 取银黄胶囊 20 粒，共 17 份，将各份样品分别置于三角瓶中密封。除 0 号瓶外，其余 16 瓶分为 4 组，每组 4 瓶，各瓶放于 50、60、70、80℃ 恒温烘箱中，按各设定时间取出，放入干燥器中冷却至室温，备用。

（2）色谱条件 高效液相色谱柱 C18（250mm×4.6mm，5μm）；流动相乙腈 -0.4% 磷酸水溶液（12∶88）；流速 0.5ml/min；柱温 25℃；检测波长 327nm。

（3）标准曲线制备 精密称取绿原酸对照品适量，置棕色量瓶中，加 50% 甲醇溶解，稀释至刻度，制成绿原酸对照品溶液（0.12mg/ml）。分别精密量取对照品溶液 1.0，2.0，3.0，4.0，5.0ml，置 10ml 容量瓶中，加流动相稀释至刻度，摇匀，按上述色谱条件各进样 10μl，记录峰面积。以浓度（C）为横坐标，峰面积（A）为纵坐标，以最小二乘法进行线性回归，得回归方程。

（4）供试品溶液制备 取上述三角瓶中银黄胶囊 10 粒内容物，研细，约取 0.2g，精密称定，置 25ml 容量瓶中，加入适量甲醇，超声处理 20 分钟，放冷，加甲醇至刻度，摇匀，0.45μm 微孔滤膜过滤，取续滤液，即为供试品溶液。

（5）样品含量测定 精密量取供试品溶液 10μl 注入色谱仪，记录峰面积，计算含量。

【数据处理】

（1）数据记录于表 20-1。以零时刻含量为 100%，求得各对应时间点的药物相对含量（%）。

表 20-1　银黄胶囊恒温加速试验数据表

温度 /℃	时间 /h	相对含量 /%	lg$C$	回归方程	K
50	0				
	8				
	16				
	24				
	32				
60	0				
	2				
	4				
	8				
	16				
70	0				
	1				
	2				
	4				
	8				
80	0				
	1				
	2				
	3				
	4				

（2）时间 t 与相对含量的对数 $\lg C$ 取直线回归，求得各温度下的直线方程，根据直线方程的斜率求得各试验温度下的反应速度常数 K 值。（如为一级反应可按下列公式计算）

$$K = -\frac{2.303}{t} \times \lg\frac{C_0}{C_t} \tag{20-1}$$

（3）根据表 20-1 的各温度下的 K 值，用 $\lg K$ 和 $1/T$ 作图，得直线方程，外推可求得室温 $25\,^\circ\mathrm{C}$（$T=273+25$）时的 K（$25\,^\circ\mathrm{C}$）值，再求出室温下药物的有效期与半衰期。

$$t_{0.9} = \frac{0.1054}{K_{25\,^\circ\mathrm{C}}} \tag{20-2}$$

$$t_{1/2} = \frac{0.693}{K_{25\,^\circ\mathrm{C}}} \tag{20-3}$$

【注意事项】加速试验温度一般至少取 4 个，每个温度需要做 4 次以上的取样分析，以保证回归方程结果准确性。

题库

思考题

1. 经典恒温加速试验法预测银黄胶囊药物有效期的原理和实验步骤是什么？

2. 本实验采用高效液相色谱法测定药物的含量，除了此法还有哪些方法可以测定药物的含量？

3. 影响本次实验结果准确性的关键操作有哪些？

4. 从制剂稳定性角度考虑，银黄胶囊在临床应用中应注意哪些问题？

Experiment 20　The Classical Isothermal Accelerated Test for Drug Stability

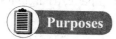 **Purposes**

1. To master the method of the classical isothermal accelerated test to predict valid period and half-life of Yinhuang Capsules.

2. To familiar with the items and methods of pharmaceutical preparation stability assessment.

3. To understand the factors that affect the stability of the pharmaceutical preparations and the stabilization method.

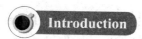 **Introduction**

1. The drug stability refers to the degree to which the chemical, physical and biological properties of the pharmaceutical preparations have altered during preparation, storage, transportation and administration. The stability experiment is to investigate the dynamic of the bulk drug or drug preparations over time under the influence of formulation factors (pH, ionic strength, excipients, etc.) and external factors (temperature, humidity, light, etc.). Provide scientific evidences for the production, packaging, storage and transportation of the drug. Determine the validity of the drug by the experiment. It is of great significance to ensure the safety and effectiveness of clinical application of drugs.

2. The stability test methods include three types: comparative test, sample observation test and accelerated test. The comparative test is generally used for the design of the formulation and the preparation procedure. The sample observation method and the accelerated test method are mostly used for the prediction of the validity of medicine.

3. The evaluation indicators of stability test usually choose the active or index ingredients of the preparation which are unstable under certain conditions (temperature, light, humidity). The determination method should be sensitive and accurate, which can reflect the variation of the concentration (content) of the index components during the accelerated test. The results should reflect the drug stability.

4. Accelerated stability testing for pharmaceutical preparations can be performed based on the principle of chemical kinetics. It can speed up the progress and shorten the testing time. The methods include classic isothermal test, simple test, empirical test and step nonisothermal test.

5. The principle of the classical isothermal testing based the Arrhenius exponential law. According to the principle of chemical kinetics, the samples are placed in thermostatic oven at different temperatures, and samples are obtained at regular intervals to assess the concentration at each temperature and time duration. Then time for the sample to decompose to a certain degree at room temperature could be reckoned by the regression equation. This method can be used for formulation screening, process

improvement, and validity prediction, but the analysis workload is large. The experimental protocol is as follows: ① Choose the temperature points and perform the accelerated test. ② Make sure the reaction order. ③ Find the K value of each test temperature. ④ Plot $\lg K$ against $1/T$ or make linear regression; ⑤ Calculate K value at room temperature (25°C). ⑥ Calculate the term validity $t_{0.9}$ and half-life $t_{1/2}$ at room temperature.

Equipments and Materials

1. Equipments　HPLC, analytical balance, ultrasonic extractor, volumetric flask, pipette, triangular flask, thermostatic oven, dryer.

2. Materials　Yinhuang Capsules, chlorogenic acid reference substance, acetonitrile (chromatographic grade), methanol, phosphoric acid, ultrapure water.

Experimental Procedures

Isothermal Accelerated Testing for Yinhuang Capsules

【Protocol】

(1) Sample processing　Take 20 capsules of Yinhuang Capsules and divide into 17 shares. Place each share in a triangle bottle and seal it. Except for No. 0 bottle, the remaining 16 bottles are divided into 4 groups, each of which has 4 bottles. Bottles are first placed in thermostatic ovens at 50, 60, 70, 80°C, respectively, and then are taken out at each set time point. All samples are put into a dryer and cooled to room temperature for later use.

(2) Chromatographic conditions　HPLC column C18 (250mm × 4.6mm, 5μm); mobile phase acetonitrile–0.4% phosphoric acid solution (12:88); flow rate 0.5ml/min; column temperature 25°C; detection wavelength 327nm.

(3) Preparation of standard curve　Precisely weight an appropriate amount of chlorogenic acid reference substance. Place it in a brown volumetric flask, add 50% methanol to make fully dissolution, and dilute to scale to make a chlorogenic acid reference solution (0.12mg/ml). Precisely transfer 1.0ml, 2.0ml, 3.0ml, 4.0ml, 5.0ml of the reference solution into a 10ml volumetric flask, and dilute to scale by adding mobile phase, mix well, and inject 10μl of each sample following the above chromatographic conditions. The peak area of each sample is record. Setting the concentration (C) as the abscissa and the peak area (A) as the ordinate, the linear regression was performed by the least square method to obtain the regression equation.

(4) Preparation of testing solution　Take the contents of ten Yinhuang Capsules from the above-mentioned triangular bottles and grind them down. Accurately weight about 0.2g of content and place it in a 25ml volumetric flask. Add an appropriate amount of methanol and sonicate for 20 min, cool down. Add methanol to scale and mix well. The solution is filtered through a 0.45μm microporous filter and take the subsequent filtrate as the testing solution.

(5) Sample determination　Precisely take 10μl of each test solution and inject it into the chromatograph instrument. Record the peak area and calculate the concentration of each sample.

【Data processing】

(1) Data records　As shown in the Table 20–1, the drug concentration at time zero was set as 100% and the relative concentration (%) of the samples at each corresponding time point was calculated.

Table 20-1　The data of isothermal accelerated testing for Yinhuang Capsules

Temperature/°C	Time/h	Relative concentration/%	lg$C$	Regression equation	K
50	0				
	8				
	16				
	24				
	32				
60	0				
	2				
	4				
	8				
	16				
70	0				
	1				
	2				
	4				
	8				
80	0				
	1				
	2				
	3				
	4				

(2) Take the linear regression of time t and the logarithm of relative concentration lg$C$ to fit the linear equations at each temperature and obtain the reaction rate constant K at each test temperature according to the slope of the linear equations. (The following equation can be employed to calculate K when it is a first-order reaction).

$$K=-\frac{2.303}{t}\times \lg \frac{C_0}{C_t} \tag{20-1}$$

(3) According to the K values at various temperatures in the Table 20-1, the lg$K$ and $1/T$ can be used to plot the linear equation, which is extrapolated to obtain the K (25°C) value at room temperature 25°C ($T = 273 + 25$). Then the half-life and validity term of the drug at room temperature can be calculated.

$$t_{0.9}=\frac{0.1054}{k_{25°C}} \tag{20-2}$$

$$t_{1/2}=\frac{0.693}{k_{25°C}} \tag{20-3}$$

【Considerations】The temperature points of accelerated testing are at least four. Each temperature point needs to be sampled four times or above to ensure the accuracy of the regression equation.

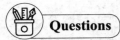

Questions

1. What is the principle and experimental procedure of the classical isothermal accelerated testing to predict the validity term of Yin-huang capsules?

2. This experiment uses high-performance liquid chromatography to determine the content of drugs. In addition to this method, what other methods can be used?

3. What are the key steps that affect the accuracy of the experiment?

4. From the perspective of drug stability, what sorts of issues should be pay attention to when use Yinhuang Capsules in clinic?

实验二十一 综合性实验与设计性实验

PPT

实验目的

1. **掌握** 制剂工艺设计的原则和步骤。
2. **熟悉** 正交试验设计及制剂工艺优选的常用方法。
3. **了解** 以二丁颗粒为例，了解制剂的质控指标与检查方法、制剂稳定性考察方法。

实验提要

1. 实验步骤

（1）确定处方

（2）选择剂型

（3）优化制备工艺（提取、分离、纯化、浓缩、干燥等）

（4）确定制剂成型工艺（优选辅料）

（5）质量控制与稳定性考察

2. 剂型的选择 以临床需要、药物性质等为依据，以毒性小、剂量小、疗效高且方便服用等为目标，通过文献调研及预试验确定。

3. 制备工艺的优化 通过文献查阅，根据处方功效，结合处方药物有效成分的理化性质及药理作用，优化提取、分离、纯化、浓缩工艺，设计合理的制备工艺路线，选择适宜的评价指标。针对可能影响制剂质量的因素，采用正交设计、均匀设计、响应曲面设计等方法，结合评价指标，优选合理的制备工艺条件，制备质量稳定的半成品。

4. 制剂成型工艺的优化 根据剂型、半成品性质等选择适宜的辅料，确定制剂成型工艺。

5. 质量控制与稳定性考察 在《中国药典》及相关行业标准指导下，进行制剂质量检查及稳定性考察。

实验器材

1. **仪器** 天平、烧杯、烧瓶、颗粒筛、烘箱等。
2. **试药** 紫花地丁、半边莲、蒲公英、板蓝根、蔗糖、糊精等。

实验操作步骤

（一）二丁颗粒的制备

【处方】

紫花地丁	250g
半边莲	250g

蒲公英	250g
板蓝根	250g
辅料适量	

【制法】 以上四味，加水煎煮两次，第一次 2 小时，第二次 1.5 小时，合并煎煮液，滤过，滤液浓缩、干燥，加入辅料适量，混匀，制成颗粒，干燥，制成 200g，即得。

实验流程图如图 21-1 所示。

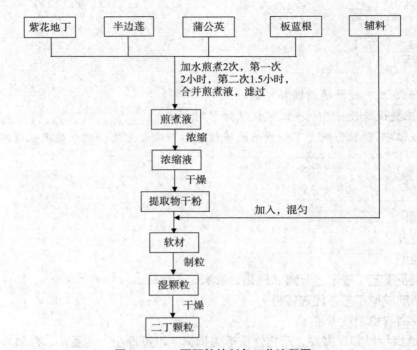

图 21-1 二丁颗粒的制备工艺流程图

【性状】 本品为棕褐色的颗粒；味甜、微苦；或味微甜、微苦（无蔗糖）。

【功能与主治】 清热解毒。用于火热毒盛所致的热疖痈毒、咽喉肿痛、风热火眼。

【用法与用量】 开水冲服。一次 1 袋，一日 3 次。

【规格】 每袋装（1）20g　（2）4g（无蔗糖）

（二）优选制备方法

1. 提取工艺优选　二丁颗粒可以水为溶剂，采用煎煮法提取药材。工艺条件优选可以煎煮次数、煎煮时间、加水量为因素，结合生产实际选择三个水平，以浸出物量、秦皮乙素含量为考核指标，选用 $L_9(3^4)$ 正交表进行正交试验。试验因素水平见表 21-1。

表 21-1　二丁颗粒提取工艺的因素水平表

水平	加水量（倍）	煎煮时间（小时）	煎煮次数（次）
1	10	0.5	1
2	20	1	2
3	30	1.5	3

对实验结果进行方差分析，确定最佳提取工艺条件，并按该工艺条件进行提取。

2. 成型工艺确定　根据提取物的性状及现有的制粒器械，通过试验确定辅料品种、用量及颗粒成型工艺。

3. **工艺验证** 按上述工艺条件制备二丁颗粒供质量检查及稳定性考察用。

（三）质量检查

1. **外观** 颗粒均匀，色泽一致，无吸潮、软化、结块、潮解等现象。

2. **水分** 照《中国药典》2020年版水分测定法（通则0832）测定，除另有规定外，水分不得超过8.0%。

3. **溶化性** 取供试品10g（中药单剂量包装取1袋），加热水200ml，搅拌5分钟，立即观察，可溶颗粒应全部溶化或轻微混浊。

4. **粒度** 取单剂量包装的5袋或多剂量包装的1袋，称定重量，置药筛内过筛。过筛时，筛保持水平状态，左右往返，边筛动边拍打3分钟。取不能通过一号筛和能通过五号筛的颗粒及粉末，称定重量，计算其所占比例不得超过15.0%。

5. **装量差异** 单剂量包装的供试品取10袋，除去包装，分别精密称定每袋内容物重量，求出每袋内容物的装量与平均装量。每袋装量与平均装量相比较（凡无含量测定的供试品或有标示装量的供试品，每袋装量应与标示装量比较），超出装量差异限度的供试品不得多于2袋，并不得有1袋超出装量差异限度1倍。

6. **微生物限度** 照《中国药典》2020年版进行检查，应符合规定。

7. **含量测定** 采用高效液相色谱法测定秦皮乙素的含量。

（四）稳定性考察

可采用恒温加速试验，考察二丁颗粒的稳定性。将颗粒剂分装于小瓶内，密封后置不同温度的恒温箱中，试验温度可根据预实验结果确定（如60℃、70℃、80℃、90℃等）。间隔一定时间取样，测定秦皮乙素的含量，利用化学动力学原理预测二丁颗粒在室温下的有效期。

思考题

1. 如何确定二丁颗粒的提取工艺和制剂工艺？

2. 正交试验设计的步骤是什么？它主要应用于哪些方面？

3. 本实验中颗粒的制备方法有哪些？应注意哪些问题？

题库

Experiment 21　Comprehensive and Designing Experiment

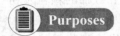

Purposes

1. To master the principles and steps of designing preparation process.

2. To be familiar with the common methods of orthogonal test design and preparation process optimization.

3. To understand the quality control indicators and inspection methods of the preparations, and the methods of examining the stability of the preparations by taking the Erding Granules as an example.

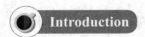

Introduction

1. Experimental procedures

(1) Determination of prescriptions

(2) Determination of dosage forms

(3) Optimization of the preparation process (extraction, separation, purification, concentration, desiccation, etc.)

(4) Determination of the molding process of preparation(optimize excipients)

(5) Quality control and stability experiment

2. Determination of dosage forms　It is determined by literature research and preliminary experiment, which is based on clinical needs, drug properties, etc., with the goal of low toxicity, low dose, high curative effect and convenient use.

3. Optimization of the preparation process　Through literature review, the extraction, separation, purification and concentration processes are optimized according to the prescription efficacy, combined with the physical and chemical properties and pharmacological effects of the active ingredients of the prescription drugs. The reasonable preparation process is designed, and the appropriate evaluation indexes are selected as well. In view of the factors that may affect the quality of the preparation, the orthogonal design, uniform design, response surface design and other methods are applied. The reasonable preparation process conditions are selected to prepare the semi-finished products with stable quality combined with the evaluation index.

4. Determination of the molding process of preparation　Select suitable excipients and determine the preparation molding process according to dosage forms, semi-finished product properties.

5. Quality control and stability experiment　Carry out the inspection of quality and stability of the preparation under the guidance of the *Chinese Pharmacopoeia* and related industry standards.

Equipments and Materials

1. **Equipments**   Balance, beaker, flask, sieve, oven, etc.
2. **Materials**   Violae Herba, Lobelia Chinensis Herba, Taraxaci Herba, Isatidis Radix, sucrose, dextrin, etc.

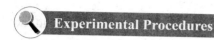

Experimental Procedures

（Ⅰ）Preparation of Erding Granules

【Formula】

Violae Herba	250g
Lobelia Chinensis Herba	250g
Taraxaci Herba	250g
Isatidis Radix	250g
Pharmaceutical adjuncts	q.s.

【Preparation】Decoct the above four herbs with water twice, 2 hours for the first time and 1.5 hours for the second time, and then mix the decoctions together. With Other processes including filtering, concentrating decoction, drying, adding appropriate amount of pharmaceutical adjuncts, uniform mixing, making granules and the second time of drying, 200g of granules is made.

Experiment flow chart (Figure 21–1):

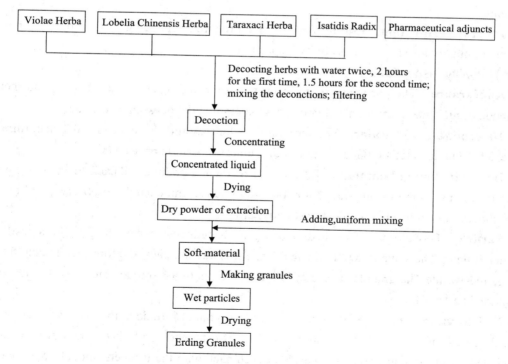

Figure 21–1   Preparation procedure of Erding Granules

【Characters】This product is brown granules; taste sweet, slightly bitter; or taste slightly sweet, slightly bitter (No sucrose).

【Functions and Indications】To remove toxic heat.For hot furuncle carbuncle, sore throat, hot eyes caused by hot poisoning.

【Usage and Dosage】1 pack, 3 times a day, taken with boiled water.

【Specification】20g or 4g (No sucrose) per bag.

(Ⅱ) Optimization of the Preparation Process

1. Optimization of extraction process Erding Granules can be extracted with water by decoction. The conditions of optimization are preferably determined by factors such as the times and duration of decoctions, and the amount of water added.

Three levels are selected according to the actual conditions, and the content of the extract and the Aesculetin are the assessment indexes. The orthogonal test is performed according to the orthogonal table $L_9(3^4)$. The level and factors of the test are shown in the Table 21-1.

Table 21-1 Factors and levels in extraction process of Erding particles

Level	Water addition	Decoction Duration/h	Decoction times
1	10	0.5	1
2	20	1	2
3	30	1.5	3

The optimum extraction conditions are determined by variance analysis of the experimental results, and extract by the conditions.

2. Determination of the molding process of preparation According to the character of the extract and granulator, the type of excipient, dosage and granule forming process are determined by experiments.

3. Process verification Erding particles are prepared according to the above technological conditions for quality inspection and stability inspection.

(Ⅲ) Quality Inspection

1. Appearance The particles are uniform, the color and luster are consistent, and there is no phenomenon of moisture absorption, softening, agglomeration, deliquescent and so on.

2. Determination of water The moisture content should not exceed 8.0% according to the moisture determination method (General rule 0832), unless otherwise provided.

3. Determination of Solubility Take 10g of medicinal granules (1 pack for granules presented in single dose) and 200ml of hot water, stir for five minutes, immediately to observe, and the soluble granules should be completely dissolved or slightly turbid.

4. Particle Take 5 packs of single dose or 1 pack of multidose, weigh the granules and sift through the medicine sieve. The sieve is kept horizontal while it is moving back and forth, with being flapped for 3 minutes meanwhile.The granules and powders which cannot pass through sieve No.1 and sieve No.5 are no more than 15.0%.

5. Weight variation Take 10 packs of medicinal granules, remove the packages, and weigh the individual content of each pack. Compare the weight of each pack with the average weight calculated (if no labeled weight is stated,compare weight of each pack with the labelled amount). Not more than 2 packs in weight variation exceed the weight variation limit above and no one bag shall exceed by 1 times.

6. Microbial limit Comply with the requirements stated under microbial limit test (ChP 2020).

7. Content determination Determine the content of aesculetin by HPLC.

（Ⅳ）Stability Experiment

The stability of the Erding Granules can be investigated by a constant temperature acceleration test. The granules are packed in a small bottle, and the temperature can be determined according to the preliminary experiment results (for example, 60℃, 70℃, 80℃, 90℃, etc.). The content of aesculetin is measured at a certain time, and the period of validity of the Erding Granules at room temperature is predicted by the principle of chemical kinetics.

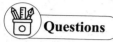

Questions

1. How to determine the extraction process and preparation process of Erding Granules?

2. What are the steps of orthogonal experimental design?

3. What are the preparation methods of granules in this experiment? What should be paid attention to?